My Marmoirs:
The True Story of a Head on a Stick

A Year-Long Journey to Beat Breast Cancer

Marcie Adams Nolan

Printed in Canada

ISBN 978-0-9811879-0-7

PRO4 22 04 09

Library and Archives Canada Cataloguing in Publication

Nolan, Marcie E., 1973-
    My marmoirs : the true story of a head on a stick / Marcie E. Nolan.

ISBN 978-0-9811879-0-7

    1. Nolan, Marcie E., 1973- --Health. 2. Breast--Cancer--Patients--Ontario-
- Guelph--Biography. I. Title.

RC280.B8N625 2009   362.196'994490092   C2009-901544-7

Praise for *Head on a Stick*

"It's a wonderful account of a tough, tough ordeal. Marcie certainly has a great sense of humour… and a way of making you feel you know the people in her life."

- Anne Lotz

"It is both enlightening and heartbreaking."

- Ruth Adams

"As we walk this journey with Marcie, many emotions surface in the writing - tears, anger, and especially humour. A very enjoyable read that any cancer patient will be able to relate to. Marcie has a way of making readers want to keep turning the pages. I was laughing, crying, remembering…YOU MADE IT! This book is great! God has truly blessed you."

- Dorothy Adams
(Mom)

"Wow! Loved it, couldn't put it down… read till almost midnight… cried, laughed, emoted… enjoyed it thoroughly."

- David Durbin

"The book is fabulous! I love it! I have cried and laughed and have gotten a much better insight as to what Marcie was really going through."

- Deb Young

"I LOVED reading this book… I am totally addicted, it is so good! Thank you for sharing your experiences, thank you, thank you. I have read the entire thing in two days and I think it's fabulous: your humour, your fear, everything comes out and is totally 'you'. Well done. It really made me feel like I lived all of those moments right there with you. I laughed out loud!"

- Tracy Manchen

"Marcie's writing is so calm, and so honest… Her sense of humour had me smiling all the way through, and I know it's what has kept her strong throughout this terrifying ordeal… I think she has the makings of a story that many other cancer patients need to read to maintain their own sense of self; the mental personality certainly becomes stronger when the physical personality is adapting to all of these changes. Marcie really is incredible, isn't she? I don't know if I could be so strong. She's in my prayers every single day."

- Laurel Karry

"WOW."

- Karin Moir

"I'll hate you in the morning! I had planned to go to bed early to nip this cold in the bud…but when I started reading your book I just couldn't stop! It's WONDERFUL! Your tone is amazing! I was so disappointed when it ended…I can hardly wait for the next installment!"

- Donna Gardner

"I finished The Marmoirs and Marcie really does have a natural gift for writing. Not only does she get this fantastic outlet for her frustration and thoughts and anger and fear and hopes, etc, but she also gets to create something that other people can enjoy and relate to and find helpful."

- Mary K. Nolan

"A story that tugs at your emotional heartstrings, while also making you laugh. A wonderful blend of hard truth and humour. Mar was already an inspiration to me before I read the book, after reading it, I admire her even more for her strength and determination. I consider Mar one of the most influential people in my life."

- Susan Rice, cousin and friend

"This book is awesome."

- Heather Harwood

"Marcie Nolan sticks her head-and her heart- out in her autobiographical book 'Head On A Stick'. You'll cry, sigh, laugh and be left wondering how she had the strength to carry on. Whether a breast cancer survivor or not, this is a must read. We're all affected by cancer. Marcie tells us how."

- Cheryl Van Ooteghem,
Principal, Sir Isaac Brock Public School

"I never knew that having breast cancer could be so hilarious! This book is a rip-roaring romp through breasts and chemotherapy!"

- Sarah Welstead

"From the devastation of diagnosis, Marcie Nolan led her life with courage and determination to become a cancer-free being again. Marcie's story is gut wrenching, daring and profound and intricately woven with clever humour. "My Marmoirs: A Year Long Journey to Beat Breast Cancer" quickly pulls in and allows the reader to gain insight into Marcie's truly remarkable battle with breast cancer."

- Monica Peirson-Durbin

"Your use of humour amidst the seriousness of your experience placed me in the front seat of the most awesome, yet terrifying, roller coaster I have ever been on. What sheer joy and heart-thumpin' 'Calgon, take me away!' feelings I experienced after reading the first pages of your book. Every word stimulated my imagination. Your work is thought provoking, extremely honest and authentic. Thank you for inspiring me and others to go beyond what is comfortable…to reach our highest level of potential."

- Yasmin Thomas-Dickey

This book is dedicated to all of the people whose lives have been forever changed by a breast cancer diagnosis.

It is for the pink angels above us and the pink warriors among us.

May we all stay strong together and never give up the fight.

Contents

Contents

Contents

Foreword

As a Physician, I am equally blessed and challenged by my interactions with the general public. To have the opportunity to share the joy of birth, to witness the sense of inner calm when reassurance is given, and to humbly accept the gratitude of those in your care when definitive action alleviates a healthcare problem is an experience few individuals are intimate with.

In stark contrast, the harsh reality of informing patients of possible life altering illnesses is both emotionally and physically draining upon a Physician. Grave news is rarely conveyed well by Physicians and this responsibility is never relished.

It was in both of these capacities that I became a willing participant in the care of Marcie Nolan. I was responsible for her care during her pregnancy, labour and delivery, while at the same time providing strength and emotional support while she dealt with her diagnosis of breast cancer.

Join with me as Marcie narrates her emotional kaleidoscope of battling a potentially life-threatening cancer while concurrently experiencing the exuberance of giving birth to her second daughter. You will tearfully rejoice while reading Marcie's self-deprecating humour and experience her courage, hope and despair while witnessing the endless support of her family and friends and the strength of her beliefs. Marcie wages her battle with cancer within the sometimes inhumane medical bureaucracy in a way that is both insightful and humbling.

This book is a must read for all, but will be especially valuable for Healthcare Professionals. To play witness to the emotional turmoil of the inner workings of a patient's psyche while she struggles to maintain her identity as an individual, as a wife, as a Mother, and as a Mother-to-be, will help us all to become more compassionate. Marcie is a true inspiration to all who seek to overcome life's obstacles, including the complexities of the illness called 'cancer'.

Gordon AD Fraser, MD

Prologue

In the beginning...

I never ever answer my phone. Ask anyone who knows me. Never. My friends already have their voicemail messages composed in their heads while my phone is ringing. I love people, I just can't talk to them on the phone. I've often wondered what it is about the phone ringing that makes my heart race and my upper lip perspire. Well, on April 28, 2005, I got my answer. Or a damn good theory, at least. Here's my story.

I was 32 years old. I was seven months pregnant with my second child. My daughter, Bryn, was just over two and a half years old. My husband loved me and I adored him. We had recently bought our first house; a beautiful house of our own in a great neighbourhood. We even had a cozy little fenced backyard full of lovely plants, flowers and enough room for our kids to run around with their friends. I was an elementary school teacher at a public school in the city where I taught French as a Second Language. I had a close group of friends to spend time with. Life was good. Life was really, really good. And then I answered my stinking phone.

"Marcie? It's Dr. MacGillivray calling. Who's there with you right now?"

Have you ever been really scared? So scared you couldn't speak? Have you ever felt so terrified that it seemed as though there was a lump in your throat? A *big* one? Me too, only it started in my right breast. The lump, I mean. Months later, as I listened to my doctor tell me news that would change my life forever, that lump moved into my throat.

"Marcie. You have breast cancer. Blah, blah, blah…" Okay, I admit that those may not have been her exact words (well, not the blah part), but after hearing the word cancer, the rest of that conversation was lost on me.

If only I hadn't answered my phone, I'd have dodged that bullet. Too late.

Chapter 1:
Finding the Lump

I did not *see that coming*

Here's a lovely image for you: me, in the shower, at about five months pregnant. I was much bigger than at that point in my first pregnancy. I remember the first time around thinking how exciting it would be to finally start wearing maternity clothes. Here I had this amazing secret but no one could tell from looking at me.

The second time around was a whole other story. This time I knew I had nine long months to get fat, angry, and uncomfortable. Why not wait a while for the fun to begin? So, there I was, in the shower, in all my pregnant glory.

As I absent-mindedly soaped up my armpit (there's another, even better, image for you) I distinctly remember the feeling of terror. The feeling of a large, hard lump in my right breast. Not the kind of lump you'd have to fish around for. Not the kind that you feel and say to yourself, "Hmm, that's odd. It's probably nothing". It was the kind of lump that sends a chill down your spine because suddenly you *know*. You may not even know yet what it is that you know, but you are certain of something.

At that moment, I pushed my gut feeling deep, deep down and began reasoning with myself. It's amazing what we're willing to believe, even from ourselves, when we really want to. "I'm pregnant. It's probably a blocked milk duct. Yes, I'm sure that's it. I'll call the doctor and set up an appointment, just to be sure."

"Yes, there's definitely something there that we need to check out," said my family doctor, Dr. Doug Choong, as his fingers found the hard mass. He explained that the chances were relatively low that this would turn out to be anything to worry about. Especially given my age. Still, being the amazing doctor that he is, and being aware of my strong family history of breast cancer, he would not send me home without further investigation. I was pregnant, of course, which ruled out the mammogram option, so he referred me to the Guelph Imaging Centre to have an ultrasound of my right breast. "Better to be safe than sorry." I agreed.

Driving home from my doctor's appointment, I remember thinking to myself how much better I felt. I had been proactive, had gone to see my doctor right away, and we were taking action. Much better than assuming it was nothing (even though it was *definitely* nothing). It's nice to be taken seriously. Even though it was nothing (did I mention that already?).

So, my denial ran deep. What can I say?

Chapter 2:
The Breast Ultrasound

Looking for lumps in all the wrong places

There I was, driving to the medical centre to get my breast ultrasound and wondering how in the world this lump had taken over my life. My breast *and* my life. A week ago the most exciting thing in my world was the baby growing inside me. I couldn't get enough of *that* lump. This new development had me reeling. Some things you just don't see coming.

I was about 5-1/2 months pregnant by the time I had an appointment for the ultrasound. Not a fun ultrasound to see my baby moving and kicking. No, this was altogether different. On some level, I believe that it was on that drive that I first felt a hint of realization that I had taken my good health for granted for many years.

I walked into the large waiting room and got in line. While waiting for the receptionist, I couldn't help but wonder what everyone else was doing there. I know it's not just me. We all do this. You look around at people, and try to tell from their facial expressions how sick they are or what life altering experiences they're dealing with.

Then you start to wonder what others are thinking about *you*. Here was this young, pregnant woman waiting for an ultrasound. Hmm, I might have been able to fly under the radar if it weren't for the look of abject terror I'm sure was glued to my face. Most happy, healthy pregnant moms are glowing. If I, at that point, was glowing, it was only because of the bright shade of green I had turned.

When it was my turn, I handed my health card to the flustered lady at the front desk. Even though it was very early in the morning, no later than 8:30 a.m., she was clearly frazzled and watching the clock for lunch.

It appeared to be clean-up day. There were piles of boxes and files everywhere behind the desk and several women were desperately trying to find Mrs. "So-and-So's" file. It looked like a nightmare. What a relief I was only there for a breast ultrasound, not to do temp work.

The rest of my wait passed uneventfully. I alternated between pretending to read my novel and looking around at the other people sitting nearby. When my name was called, my heart skipped a beat, just one, and then I was fine. I followed a young woman to the change area where I was instructed to take off my shirt and bra, and to put on the gown that was sitting on the bench in the cubicle.

I did as directed and met the woman in an ultrasound room across the hall. She had me lie on my back and open my gown. Thankfully, I was in the care of a real people-person. Throughout the procedure, we talked about our children, my pregnancy, the weather. I was quite relaxed by the time we finished.

I was asked to sit up and wait a few minutes while the technician checked the photos. She wanted to make sure she had all the shots she needed before I changed back into my clothes.

The moment the technician walked back into the room followed by a middle-aged man in a white lab coat, a voice inside my head screamed. He introduced himself as Dr. "Something-Or-Other", a radiologist. He had taken a look at my ultrasound images and was concerned about the lump he saw.

He explained in a very sombre tone that there appeared to be blood moving into and out of the mass. Apparently, that's a bad thing. It signalled some kind of interaction between the mass and the rest of my body. This, too, was bad.

If you are a doctor reading this and thinking to yourself, "*No*, that's not how it works" or something along those lines, I apologize. As a lay person, medical jargon is not my forte, especially in a situation where my mind has already gone into panic mode. I am simply telling it as I remember it, in the terms that made sense to me at the time. There is every possibility that much of what I recall about any medical explanation given to me is complete crap.

The radiologist said that it could have something to do with me being pregnant. It was possible. His face showed that it was an unlikely possibility, but I have to give the guy credit for throwing me a bone.

Still, he asked the technician how quickly she could send the ultrasound images to my family doctor and she replied that, with it being a Friday, she could get them there early the following week.

When the man in the white lab coat replied, "I want you to fax them to his office today," I knew my fears were justified. I was told to call as soon as I got home and make an appointment to see my family doctor. Since he assists in surgeries at the hospital on Fridays, he does not have any office hours. I would call him first thing Monday morning.

I went back into the small change cubicle, got dressed and neatly folded my gown. I set it in the small hamper beside the bench. I sat for a long time. And I cried. I wept quietly to myself and felt, suddenly, what it might feel like to learn that you have cancer. It must feel something like this. That sinking, heavy feeling.

It may be hard to believe, but up until that very moment I had not considered the possibility that I might have cancer. Not once. Not really, anyway. I knew the tests were all to make sure I didn't have cancer. But not to determine that I *did* have cancer. That was an outcome I hadn't really considered.

You know the expression "long weekend"? Well, I sure had one after that ultrasound. Not the kind of long weekend in which you spend an extra day or two with your loved ones, eating turkey and pumpkin pie, but the other kind. The kind that goes on and on and on and on, even though it technically has the same number of hours as a regular weekend.

Why is it that some weekends, the long holiday kind, can fly by so quickly and yet others, the regular kind, can creep along so painfully slowly? I believe that terror is the answer to that question. Pure, unbridled terror.

Back in Dr. Choong's office on Monday afternoon, the familiar, handsome face of my family physician calmed my nerves at once. He is the kind of man you'd like to just sit and have a coffee with. A guy you'd probably want to become friends with, if you met him at a party.

I always thought that doctors were scary. So smart. So powerful. So intimidating. Dr. Choong is very smart and very powerful, but so down to earth that I can (and have) talked to him about absolutely anything, no matter how big or small, how embarrassing or personal.

We sat in his office for a long time, long enough for me to really ask my questions without feeling rushed. Dr. Choong answered my questions honestly, in enough detail to help put my mind at ease. He never once tried to tell me it was absolutely nothing, or that I was being paranoid. He simply explained some realistic possibilities and let me know that he would be sending me to the experts to look more closely at the lump so we could find out what we were dealing with. I liked knowing that "we" were on the same team. It was reassuring to know that, whatever happened, he would walk me through it one step at a time.

Leaving Dr. Choong's, my mind was in a much better place. I knew that he had referred me to a general surgeon in the city. She was, he assured me, an amazing surgeon with a great bedside manner. She was a young woman herself and understood women and their concerns, not that Dr. Choong didn't.

Dr. MacGillivray was, in fact, "The Breast Lady" in Guelph. I would go and await The Breast Lady's call. It would all be fine in the end.

Chapter 3:
The Needle Biopsy

Not to put too fine a point on it

Next stop, the office of Dr. Jean MacGillivray, General Surgeon, Breast Lady and overall damn good person. It takes a special doctor to be able to meet someone, a total stranger, and make her feel comfortable enough to let you feel her up within minutes.

We chatted about this and that and before I knew it, I'd had a needle biopsy and was getting dressed to go home. I should probably clarify something here: I am, and have always been, really, really, really bad around all things medical. All things hospital. All things bloody. All things scary. All things... well, practically *all* things.

So, the idea of a needle biopsy was right up there with, say, giving birth without an epidural, which, by the way, I've never had the horror of experiencing but in my mind, the two are perfect equals.

The good doctor (and she *is* good) spoke to me calmly yet with a serious tone. I understood right away that, once again, I was being taken seriously, my lump was being investigated thoroughly, and that we would get answers to the "What the hell is it?" question as soon as possible. She would send off the biopsy samples and, as an extra measure of care, she was referring me to the Guelph General Hospital to have a core biopsy done.

Now, I hate to dwell on small details, but picture me if you can, having just completed a needle biopsy (which, I'll admit, sounds worse than it is, not that I'd recommend you go out and get one just so you can see for yourself) and now learning that another, *bigger*, biopsy was in my imminent future.

Not good. Bad. Really bad. Of course, being a total phony in many regards, I nodded, smiled and said something along the lines of "Thank you, Dr. MacGillivray. Thank you. Yes. That's wonderful. Thank you." Crap.

Meeting Dr. MacGillivray was just the beginning in terms of my journey toward facing my fears. OK, ultrasound: check. Needle biopsy: check. Two creepy items off my to-do list, too many others left to count. It all seemed like a lot of commotion, a lot of action, and a lot of precaution for nothing. It was definitely going to turn out to be nothing after all this fuss. Man, I couldn't wait to look back on it and laugh. Ha.

Chapter 4:
Meeting My Obstetrician

Hey baby, come here often?

Keep in mind that I was a glowing, pregnant version of myself at this time. The acne. The weight gain. The bags under my eyes. Quite a sight to behold. I know they always say a woman is at her most beautiful when she is with child, but let me beg to differ. Let's be real. I was at my hottest when I was 16, slim yet shapely, and too young to realize that I was at my peak of physical loveliness. Youth really *is* wasted on the young.

So, at the time that I was awaiting word on when my core biopsy would be performed, I was also waiting to meet my obstetrician for the first time. I had seen a different ob/gyn when pregnant the first time around and was a bit nervous to meet "the new baby guy".

My family doctor had recommended him when I had whined about not really "clicking" with my previous ob/gyn. He, "the first baby guy", had been amazing at his job, a very professional man, but I just didn't feel that certain closeness I thought was necessary. Given the personal and intimate nature of the woman-ob/gyn relationship, I just wanted to feel more at ease.

There aren't a ton of obstetricians in Guelph, so when you mention a name, there are always a lot of women who have stories to share. I spoke to some friends and asked around, hoping to get a feel for what was to come. Again, I'll remind you of my wooziness when it comes to all things medical. Having babies counts as medical, in my experience. I was nervous, to say the least, and hoped to allay my fears of the unknown before my first appointment.

"My friend's friend fired him. She couldn't stand him!" "Mine, too. What a jerk!" Gee, I'm so glad I asked.

I was sitting in a chair beside a desk in the small patient room of my new obstetrician's office. Not much to look at (the office, I mean). I had found the receptionist and the nurses really friendly, so that was a good start. Waiting. Waiting. Expecting to wait for at least an hour and a half, as I had last pregnancy.

I'd brought a good book, just to pass the time. Oh, and I had taken a plastic bottle from a basket marked with a note reading: "Please take one. Obstetrics patients should need only one bottle throughout their pregnancy. Please reuse your bottle." I wondered if the bottles were dishwasher-safe. Then I wondered if it was wrong on some level to consider putting a urine bottle in the dishwasher. Just for the record, I opted to hand wash it each time.

Enter Dr. Gord Fraser. In casual pants and a golf shirt, sandals (no socks) and a warm smile, he made direct eye contact right away. I love that. I was just thinking to myself, "I really like this guy" when he spoke. Why do men always have to do that - spoil it by talking? Kidding, kidding. He introduced himself, had a peek at my chart, which, let's be honest, only had my weight on it at that point, and started in on a well-rehearsed blurb about what to eat, not eat, do and not do to *not* get any fatter. Are you familiar with the sound a bubble makes when it bursts? Arghhh.

I left the office, drove to McDonald's and ordered a super-sized version of some combo I didn't really even want. With a diet Coke, of course. I couldn't believe he was making such a big deal about my weight. I knew it wasn't going to work out with him. No way. What kind of sadist tells a woman, a *pregnant* woman, she's *fat*? Okay, he didn't use the word "fat" per se, but that's what he meant.

I had a month to cool down before our next visit.

Chapter 5:
Back to the Obstetrician

Hit me baby, one more time

By the time I found myself driving to my next appointment, I had decided he was probably still a fine obstetrician and as long as he knew how to get the baby out, I'd let the weight stuff slide for now. I had enough on my mind and was clearly going to have to choose my battles.

I sat in the bright waiting area, plastic bottle in hand, like so many other women in the room. Nowhere else but at her obstetrician's office would a woman feel right at home holding a container of her own urine.

As always, I looked around at the various women, in all shapes, sizes and at all stages of pregnancy. I couldn't help but envy them, assuming, of course, that they were enjoying a "normal" lump-free pregnancy. They would never know from looking at me that my mind was far from my pregnancy most of the time. Until I got word, my brain had room for nothing else but constant worry.

I had had enough time to get my game plan ready for facing Dr. Fraser. I would politely listen to his schpiel about my weight. I would smile and nod. I would ask him my pregnancy-related questions. I would leave.

There was no reason to expect this man to be anything more than the one who would eventually free me of the larger of my two lumps. It is very helpful to accept certain things early on. I decided that Dr. Fraser's obsession with weight gain was the least of my worries, so I would just hear him out and not let it get to me. Why go there?

Besides, since the lump incident, and the ultrasound incident, and the biopsy incident, my appetite was shot and there was very little eating going on. Weight loss had become a reality for me, not weight gain.

Again I found myself sitting in the little patient room awaiting Dr. Fraser. I listened to voices in the hall outside the closed door. I read the outdated pamphlets on the bulletin board. I psyched up for "the weight talk". Knock knock. In poked my obstetrician's head around the partially opened door. That smile. Those eyes. I admit it's hard to stay mad at someone like him. Believe me, I tried.

Every once in a while I am lucky enough to be pleasantly surprised. This meeting, for me, was one of those occasions, maybe even the mother-of-all pleasant surprises.

Dr. Fraser, looking directly into my eyes, a bedside skill for which I have such respect, asked me how I was *feeling*. You read that right. He wanted to know how I was *feeling* since we last met. I found myself unable to hold back my true emotions, emotions I had not shared with anyone yet outside my immediate family and closest friends.

I was awaiting word on tests about a breast lump that might not be "nothing", and I was terrified. I recall holding back tears as I spoke. I can also picture the compassion in Dr. Fraser's eyes as he listened to my words.

Are you ready for the best part? He hugged me. A big, warm bear hug. It said everything to me. It said he understood I was afraid. It said I would be OK no matter what. It said he cared about me and would support me in any way he could. All that from one hug.

When I walked out of that office and into the lobby, my feet may not have been touching the ground. That may sound dramatic, but the feeling of a weight off my shoulders was very real. I had needed to put my feelings out into the world, to speak them out loud and be heard, and I never would have guessed that Dr. Fraser would have been the one on the listening end.

Since that day, my love and respect for Dr. Fraser have only grown. We have had a number of heart-to-hearts and his advice has been invaluable to me and my family on many occasions. He speaks his mind, makes me laugh and, above all, he is the one who has said all along, "You are going to be fine". Sometimes you just need to hear what you want to hear. Most of the time, I even believe him.

Chapter 6:
The Core Biopsy

Cuts like a knife

Walking through the doors of the Guelph General Hospital, I recall having a surreal, out-of-body feeling. I was on a mission, looking for the right floor, the right reception desk, the right waiting room. It was as though I were taking charge for someone who couldn't look after herself. A friend in need. Not me. If I had truly registered that I was indeed there for myself, I believe, in hindsight, that I would have run away screaming and never returned.

There I was. Waiting. Waiting. Waiting. Luckily, the receptionist had handed me some pamphlets to prepare me for my "procedure". If you ever find yourself in this, or a similar, situation, I'd like to go on record as strongly recommending you *not* prepare yourself for your "procedure". There is definitely such a thing as too much information. In my case, and in my mental state, I'm thinking Cosmo or People magazine might have been more helpful to prepare me.

While watching the clock (and checking my watch and my husband's watch, in case there was a discrepancy), I would have loved to have read all the Hollywood gossip. Nothing helps more in a time of crisis than to read about other people's problems, even if 99 percent of what we read in trashy magazines is pure fiction. After learning about Brad and Jen's split and the imminent arrival of Tom and Katie's lovechild, at least I could've comforted myself with the knowledge that my husband, sweating like a pig in the chair beside me, was *there* with me and did not belong to the Church of The Frisbee.

It's funny what you remember and forget about stressful situations. How does the brain decide what to retain and what to delete? I recall vividly that, upon hearing my name called, I looked to my left. I looked to my right. Nope, no other Marcie Adams here. I guess I'll go ahead then. It's as if I actually thought that other women named Marcie Adams were unfortunate enough to be sitting there, too, waiting for core biopsies. Poor things. That would suck.

Now is as good a time as any to bring up the whole name thing. OK, I admit it, at that point I had been married for 5-1/2 years to a wonderful man, Jeff Nolan, and I still hadn't changed my name on my health card. I had changed my name on everything else: credit cards, driver's licence, that sort of thing. Just not my health card. Which was fine, since I was so very healthy all my life.

The health card is a card you rarely use if you are fortunate enough to be in good health. Once in a blue moon, you pull it out at an appointment and say to yourself that you should really get that name changed. Then you put the card in your wallet, have a seat in the doctor's waiting room, pick up a Chatelaine from summer 2001, and become engrossed in a recipe for homemade guacamole.

Next thing you know, you've seen the doctor, driven home, prepared dinner and it's as if the health card doesn't even exist. Until your next appointment, when you pull it out and say to yourself that you should really think about getting that name changed. You get my point.

"Marcie Adams?" Again, the mind is a funny thing. I have no recollection of getting from the waiting room to the biopsy room. I'm assuming I walked there, probably with a fake, sweet smile on my face so no one around me would feel uncomfortable. Wouldn't want that.

I don't remember changing, either, but I do recall the gown I put on. A very good look. A short strappy number, with an option to wear it open in the front or back. I opted for front-opening, what with the breasts being there and all. Mental note: always shave legs before a "procedure," even if the "procedure" is being done to your breast.

I was shown to a bed - a tall, thin, creepy bed. I sat on the very edge, giving myself the illusion that I could still easily run away at any moment if I decided to. The technician was a very nice woman, calm and friendly, so we gabbed for a bit. She explained that she was going to do an ultrasound of my entire right breast, taking pictures for the hospital records. I was instructed to please lie down and open the gown.

If you recall, my last breast ultrasound did not go terribly well. So, how much worse could this one really be? It was simple and non-threatening. I believe that I had already begun the process of disconnecting from my right breast by that point. It was also becoming increasingly easy to bare my breasts when asked by perfect strangers. When this was all behind me, I should really look into wet T-shirt contests.

Immediately following the ultrasound, the radiologist came in and introduced himself. I don't remember his name, but I know he was a soft-spoken man with kind eyes. He clearly explained the steps he would be taking to perform the core biopsy. Part of my right breast was frozen and we were ready to begin.

Well, he was. I was ready to vomit. It actually didn't sound *that* bad when he went over it. I felt a slight sense of relief that at least I was there, it was going to be done and I could soon move on. Then he pulled out what I shall forever refer to as "the instrument of torture".

Picture a staple gun. A big one. Or one of those ear-piercing gadgets they use at the mall. Not good. The doctor was kind enough to "shoot" it a few times in the air so I could familiarize myself with the sound it would make when plowing into my breast flesh. Very helpful, doctor. Thank you. I guess he figured it would be better for me to be fully prepared for my "procedure". Funny, I didn't read about that part in the pamphlet.

Let me explain to you in non-medical terms what a core biopsy is, in case you are lucky enough to have never heard of such a thing until now. A core biopsy is a method of removing a plug of tissue, or several plugs if needed, for the purpose of examining it for cancer or other conditions. In my case, they were examining the tissue for cancer. The plugs are taken with the aid of an ultrasound screen so that samples from a specific site can be removed.

Sometimes we can look back on experiences or events in our lives and say "Wow, I get it now". The core biopsy experience is one of those times that I can look back on and laugh, because it all makes sense.

When the radiologist first walked into the room and introduced himself to me, he had my file in his hand. He opened it up casually and took a look inside. He said, "Oh, I see that you have a surgery date already booked for early May". Of course, I laughed and said, "No, not that I know of, at least." Hahaha.

He quickly closed my file and mumbled, "I must have the wrong file." Hahaha again. We shared a good chuckle and were ready to begin the torture, I mean, "procedure".

Soon enough I would revisit what the radiologist had said about the surgery date in May with a whole new understanding. But not yet.

The radiologist performing my biopsy took four or five samples of tissue from the lump in my right breast. He put each one in its own container to be examined. At one point he said something along the lines of, "Oh, these are good samples". How could he tell? I was proud of my tissue for being so "good". I probably thanked him, as if it were a compliment to me personally.

When my biopsy was complete, a nurse explained to me how to ice the sore spot for the next several hours. I always knew the bag of sweet peas in my freezer would come in handy. If not for a shepherd's pie, then for a makeshift icepack.

I was told that it would take about a week for the results to be available and that my surgeon would receive a copy of them and contact me. A week sounded like a long time to wait, but it was over and I was glad.

For the rest of that day, I was sore and swollen, gingerly walking to the freezer to exchange the damp peas for the frozen corn niblets and vice versa. It was, however, a great excuse to put my feet up and watch my ladies, Oprah and Ellen.

At that point in time, I was still taking my daughter to her babysitter most days, and Jeff was off to work from eight until four. It was a rare occurrence to find myself home alone with nothing to do. I read my O magazines, napped and channel-surfed until it was time to get dinner started (and by "get dinner started" I mean "decide what to have on our pizza before calling in the order"). No way was I cooking!

At the end of that long day, I recall slipping into bed, barely able to keep my eyes open. The stress of the biopsy had taken its toll and I needed to get some sleep. I had a busy day of couch-potatoing ahead and wanted to be at the top of my game.

I awoke refreshed. I had the entire day to myself with no plans, nothing pressing to be done, and I couldn't wait to hurry up and relax. Much like the day before, I watched Ellen and Oprah, flipped through the latest O magazine and dozed off whenever I felt sleepy.

At one point, I remember turning off the television and just lying on the couch listening to the silence. With a 2-1/2 year-old daughter usually running around the house, silence was generally a thing that signalled she was up to no good. This silence was different. Sweet. And then the phone rang.

"Marcie? It's Dr. MacGillivray calling. Who's there with you right now?"

Chapter 7:
Sharing My Breast Cancer Diagnosis

You may want to sit down for this

I hung up the phone, stunned. My body was reacting to the news that I had breast cancer, but my brain was not. Not yet. How could it?

No more waiting. No more hoping. No more denial (well, a bit from time to time). I can still feel my heart beating wildly, frantically. I was sweating, although I had been standing perfectly still for some time.

I cried a quick fit of hysterical tears and then pulled myself together to call my husband, my sister, my father and my best friends. Suddenly the quiet house was suffocating me.

Some people hate to worry others or to "burden" them. Clearly, I am not one of those. I called my husband, choked out the words, "You have to come home". I recall his only comment before hanging up the phone to be "Oh f@#!$".

Next, I called my sister. "Sister" is not even a strong enough word for who Shelley is, for what Shelley means to me. Of course, that was a day my sister was working at a different location, away from her office. I called the front desk, they paged her and there was no answer. I hung up, having left a high-pitched message, saying something like, "Please have her call me when she gets a minute". Then I very patiently waited for about 30 seconds. Why hadn't she called me back yet? I dialed the front desk again, and asked would they mind trying to page her again? It really was an emergency.

"Hello?" came the sound of my favourite voice. It was a question, the kind that asks, "What's wrong?" I had pulled myself together to speak to the receptionist, and that alone was a miracle. But you know how it is when you really, really love someone? It is physically impossible to keep it together when you hear their voice at a time of crisis. I'm not exactly sure what I said to her at that time. I only know that I cried for her to come and that, seemingly in an instant, she was coming through my front door, arms outstretched and silent tears falling, almost before I hung up the receiver.

Next, a call that would send shivers down any child's spine. I called my dad in London, Ontario. No child, at any age, wants to have to tell her parent that she has cancer. It is still, to this day, one of the hardest calls I've ever had to make.

I had kept my dad, Don, and step-mom, Dorothy, in the loop about the lump and the tests. I had also always stressed to them that all of the doctors felt it would turn out to be a "pregnancy thing". We were just erring on the side of caution.

As for my father, I look back now and wonder if he worried much more throughout the waiting period than it appeared. He must have. He is strong. He is the one who props us up when things get ugly. But even the strongest father is human. I can't for the life of me imagine the terror a parent would experience at the thought of an ill child, especially after having already lost his wife far too young. I give my dad credit for finding a way to keep my spirits up when, in hindsight, I can't even fathom the chaos in his own mind. He offered to come right away, and, suddenly being a young child again, I said, "Yes. Come quickly."

Finally, my best friends. Women in my age group. Young moms. Young wives. Young daughters. Young sisters. How close to home would my news hit them? In what ways would they be forever changed by this call? Did I even have the strength to tell this story over and over again to the women who meant so much to me in so many different ways?

We have all heard the expression "fair-weather friends," those friends who are there with you when things are good, when life is fun and when there is no hard work to be done, either physically or emotionally. They, too, are the friends who quickly disappear at the first sign of trouble. If it is support and a shoulder to cry on that you need, you must look beyond them. They are so far away they wouldn't hear you if you called out for them.

Well, it is true that some people just can't handle the tough times. I understand that. I really do. The thing that makes that OK, in my mind, is the fact that the friends who stayed, who rallied around me, who laughed and cried and ranted and raved with me, far outnumbered the ones who ran away.

I know now that I am blessed. I may have sensed it before, but I am ashamed to admit that it was in a "taking people for granted" sort of way. Going through this experience has shown me in a whole new way how fortunate I am to have the support of my family physician, my close family members and best friends. I have a husband who loves me deeply, flaws and all (not that there are many of those, of course!). I have my beautiful children. I have religious ministers and fellow worshippers who pray for me and with me.

In my time of need I also had e-mails, cards, gifts, letters, casseroles, kisses, flowers, and jokes-of-the-day. I had fun, friendly neighbours who mowed my lawn and shoveled my driveway and took my oldest daughter to the park so I could rest. I had work colleagues who bent over backwards to make me feel loved and supported while away from my job.

I could type all day, listing blessing after blessing and gift after gift. Not everyone in a scary situation can say they have the immense unconditional love and support around them at all times that I am thankful to have had. If all clouds have a silver lining, this one would be the opportunity to fully realize and appreciate everything and everyone I have in my life and the new perspective it provides for the future.

Chapter 8:
Telling the Neighbours

Buenos dios, neighbouritos!

Not everyone can say that their neighbours are their friends. Lots of people are "friendly" with their neighbours but would not actually call them up to hang out. We, on the other hand, are good friends with Mike and Deb Young. At the time of my cancer diagnosis, they lived right next door to us. I still remember meeting them for the first time. Shelley, Jeff and I were sitting on our upper deck in the backyard, not having completely moved in yet, when I heard a noise next door.

I stood up and looked over the fence. It was Deb and Mike, coming out to start the barbecue. I said hello and introduced myself to them. From the look on their faces, I had caught them off guard with my friendly introduction. We were technically strangers, after all. They were no doubt wondering if I was going to turn out to be that annoying neighbour who would call over the fence to them every time they went out into their yard. Well, I did turn out to be that neighbour.

The couple we bought our house from had told us that the neighbours "over there" had a little girl named Madison who was about the same age as our daughter, Bryn. We were quite excited at the thought of Bryn having someone so close to play with. Having moved from an apartment building to our first house, the idea of next-door neighbours was new to us.

At some point once we were fully moved in and getting settled, we got the girls together for a play date. They were introduced once and became fast friends instantly. They are two strong, independent little children and I believe that they each found their match in the other that day.

Time went by and Deb and I began spending more and more time together so that the girls could play. As we sat, watching Bryn and Madison form a love-hate relationship of epic proportions, we slowly got to know each other better. I began to look forward to the play dates so I could catch up with Deb. We had similar lives, senses of humour, parenting styles and attitudes. That made it very easy to sit and pass the time together while the girls were playing.

Jeff and I had been in the house for nearly a year when I was diagnosed with breast cancer. By then, it had really stopped being all about Bryn and Madison. Deb and I were friends and got together because we wanted to, not only for the girls. When I think about having to tell my closest friends about my diagnosis, Deb comes to mind immediately. She was, by that time, the first person I called to share exciting news with, the person I saw the most often and one of the people I cared most about.

In fact, not only had Deb and I become close friends, but our husbands had gotten to know each other as well. Many summer nights were spent with the four of us in one backyard or the other, having a barbecue and hanging out while the girls played in the yard. We all loved the same movies, were laid-back parents and had such fun laughing about the latest adventures of parenthood and married life in our thirties. Never a dull moment.

I had confided in Deb early on that I had found a breast lump and needed to have it tested. I had kept her posted on the biopsies. Deb knew that I was waiting for the big news. She had, at that time, already lost her best friend to cancer. Steph had fought it long and hard. Deb was devastated by the loss. So, the thought of telling her that I, too, had cancer, was impossible to even imagine.

And then it happened. I learned that I had breast cancer and Deb was one of the first people I wanted to talk to, to tell. I hadn't quite come up with the best way to say it when we ran into each other in our driveways. She was just arriving home as I was about to head out, or vice-versa, and we stopped to talk. She asked if I had heard anything yet, and I told her that I had. It was bad news. I could see in her eyes that she understood before I said it. Still, to make it real even to myself, I had to say it. I had breast cancer and would need to have a lumpectomy soon.

Deb and I had formed a very close but very interesting relationship. It had not been built on deep emotions, at least not in the sense that we sat around crying in front of each other about our problems. Neither one of us was really like that. We always ended up finding the humour in things eventually. So, we were truly close but not in a huggy, touchy-feely way.

This posed an interesting challenge, what with the cancer and all. In my mind, it was amazing just to have Mike, Deb and Madison right next door. They were good friends to us at the best of times, and they certainly made our lives easier in the worst of times. Still, when I was feeling scared, sad, angry, or volatile, I did not want to "go there" in front of Deb. It was definitely not because I felt I couldn't. I knew Deb was a safe person to fall apart in front of. I think it was more difficult because she, they, were such a part of our day-to-day lives.

Most often when we all got together, the kids were there. They may have been off doing their own thing, but they were close enough to have noticed if I fell apart. So, venting to Deb would have been tricky. I wanted to shelter both girls, Madison and Bryn, from what was happening, from what was about to happen. They were not quite three years old yet and cancer had no meaning in their worlds. I didn't want to be the one to introduce it to them.

So, Deb and I visited often and talked a lot. I told her everything that was going on but admit that, without really realizing it at the time, I put on a brave face much more often than was necessary. I wonder, looking back, if my own need to keep up a happy façade in my neighbourhood, to appear "just fine", made it harder for Deb to deal with what was happening to me and to talk to me about it, too. If I had it to do all over again (which I don't intend to have happen), I'd let Deb in more and say "Screw the façade! This really sucks!" She's strong. She could take it! When I next find myself in a crisis situation, I plan to let Deb see my ugly cry. If she doesn't bolt then, we really are friends for life!

When I returned home from the lumpectomy surgery, it was springtime. The sun was out, the grass and flowers were growing and the kids wanted to be outside playing every waking minute. I was in such pain, carrying Dana around in my belly and Bryn hanging onto me everywhere I went. Healing from a lymph node dissection was harder than I thought it would be, and being pregnant meant that I was unable to take the stronger pain medications that are usually prescribed after this sort of surgery. I ached constantly, was brought to tears regularly, but wanted desperately to keep Bryn's little life normal. I wanted to be outside playing tag, digging in the sandbox, chasing bugs. Or at least I wanted to want to. But I didn't. Truth be told, I wanted to curl up in my sick bed and stay there for as long as it took for the pain to ease up.

This is where having a friend for a neighbour, or a neighbour for a friend, came in handy. Very regularly, Deb and I would meet in our backyards to let the girls play. That spring and all summer long, Deb was like the mother of two: Madison *and* Bryn. Deb became the healthy playmate, the fun parent that I simply couldn't be. She seemed to always be aware that I was struggling with a high level of pain, and knew I was trying hard to pretend it wasn't that bad. She also always made it OK to take her help.

That summer, Deb played many roles. She was Madison's mom, Bryn's "mom", my friend, our neighbour, Jeff's saviour, a monster chasing the girls around the yard, to their delight, an airplane flying them up in the sky, a sandbox digger, a sandcastle maker, a bike- and swing-pusher, a food-sharer (thank God, or we'd all have starved) and so much more. I'm not entirely sure what we'd have done without Deb in those days, and I'd rather not even think about that. Luckily for the Nolans, she was there.

Mike, too, played a big role in getting us through the hard times. It was good for Jeff to have a guy to hang out with. Many a mild evening, we'd walk next door with a few bottles of beer in hand, for a casual, impromptu visit. Inevitably, the guys would fall into their "guy talk" (you know, movies, meat and beer) and the gals would fall into their "gal talk" (you know, making fun of our husbands while they were sitting right there, clueless). Just having a man around was helpful to Jeff. Him having a guy to talk to was also helpful to me, because it made me feel good to know he had an escape from reality so near home.

As summer turned to fall, and then winter, we awoke on more than one occasion to find that the "snow-shoveling fairy" had cleared out our driveway (I am in no way suggesting that our neighbour is a fairy of any kind!). Mike is a police officer and works shifts, sometimes getting home late at night. On those late nights, he often headed outside and shoveled both driveways. It was such a treat to wake up, look outside and see that our car had a clear path to get out. Not shovelling was one less thing to worry about, especially for Jeff since I was physically unable to do it. Most chores, inside and out, fell on Jeff's shoulders to complete. It was a huge help for us both every time Mike took one for the Nolan team.

Jeff once confided in me guiltily that he had taken a "sick" day. He had been feeling exhausted, stressed out and too drained to concentrate at the office. Instead, he had stayed home in his pyjamas all day. It was a mental health day, and much-needed. He played the guitar most of the day. As he played, he became aware of a scraping sound outside. It sounded as if it was coming from our driveway. I had taken the girls to London to visit Nana and Papa, so our car was not in the driveway as it normally would have been. Generally, as Mike knew, if our car wasn't in the driveway, we were out.

On that particular day, Mike had been shovelling his driveway and saw that no one was home at the Nolan house. It was a cold, blustery day, with the snow coming down as quickly as it was being shovelled up. Little did he know that Jeff was inside, lazing around, strumming away on his guitar with a soccer game playing on TV in the background. The sound outside was, indeed, our wonderful neighbour, Mike.

Jeff peeked out the window, saw Mike out there, freezing, shovelling our driveway, and shuffled back to his guitar and his game. No, he did not run out and admit he was home. No, he did not offer to finish it up. Let's face it, he did exactly what I would've done. He pretended no one was home. It's nice to let people help sometimes, right? Thanks, Mike.

Chapter 9:
Support from the People
of Jeff's Workplace

Fly like an Eagle

This seems like a good time to give a huge shout-out to Eagle's Flight, Incorporated.

In 2002, Jeff was fortunate enough to find employment at a consulting company in downtown Guelph. It was a company built from the ground up by a man named Phil Geldart. Phil's work and life vision, as well as his family-oriented, Christian values, appealed to Jeff immediately and we celebrated on the day he was offered a year-long contract with the company.

At that time, we had recently moved to Guelph from the Toronto area and Jeff was a frustrated, albeit dedicated, commuter, driving day after day to his office in Etobicoke. Eagle's Flight turned out to be a perfect fit for Jeff, and his job position in the newly-created Measurement department was one that he both enjoyed and found challenging.

Also at that time, we were expecting our first baby. We lived in a two-bedroom apartment right downtown (within easy walking distance to Eagle's Flight) and I was teaching at Brant Avenue Public School in Guelph. We were happy with our life and excited to try our hand at parenthood.

Skip ahead to pregnancy number two, filling in the long gap by simply assuming that all was well up until that point, which is true. Given my unexpected, untimely (not that there's really a "good time" to be diagnosed with anything ugly) breast cancer diagnosis, we suddenly found ourselves in need of help.

Thankfully, Jeff was still an employee at Eagle's Flight and Phil Geldart, the company leader, stepped up to the plate immediately upon hearing the devastating news. Phil and his employees (in all departments at all times) proved that the company's mission statement – core values and Christian family-oriented philosophies were not simply words. They were real and very much alive at Eagle's Flight.

Early on in the process, Jeff was given time off to accompany me to my many tests and appointments, several of which were in Hamilton and, therefore, took the best part of a day. Without hesitation, Jeff's boss, Christy Pettit, also approved Jeff's request to work from home as needed. He was able to drive me to every single chemotherapy treatment, sit by my side (or in a near-by cancer centre bathroom, due to his own nausea) or stay behind to be with our children in a guilt-free fashion. Not once did pressure to be at the office add an extra burden to Jeff's already broken back and spirit.

Jeff eventually applied for parental leave, and dealt with the Human Resource Department at EF for the first (and not last) time. The paperwork was completed and his two-month leave was a done deal. Again, no pressure, no guilt trips, only support and encouragement from the Measurement Team and other departments. Without Jeff at home throughout this difficult period, I'm sure I don't have to tell you what creek I'd have been up.

As the two months went on, it became evident that I was not yet ready to be the primary caregiver and homemaker. Jeff was badly needed on the home front, so back to HR he went. He returned home with an extension of parental leave that would last, in total, six months. He also returned home with flowers, cards, gifts, and well-wishing e-mails from colleagues that he had printed off to share with me.

I know you think I'm using my "artistic licence" to embellish this part of the story, but I kid you not, Jeff works for the most compassionate company we have ever heard of. That anyone has ever heard of. Upon sharing the details of Jeff's numerous and lengthy work absences with our family and friends, we have been witness to many a shocked disbeliever. No one, and I mean no one, to this day, has had a story of work support that could hold a candle to ours.

So, because I'm a bit behind (by a few years or so, give or take) in my thank-you cards, I want to take this opportunity to say "thank you" to Phil Geldart, Christy Pettit and all of Jeff's many colleagues at Eagle's Flight.

Thankyouthankyouthankyouthankyouthankyouthanky-outhankyouohso much.

Chapter 10:
Explaining Breast Cancer
to My Toddler

Once upon a time…

I had six days between my cancer diagnosis and my appointment in the operating room for a lumpectomy. What do you do with that kind of time? It was the most eerie, uncomfortable, and unreal time I have ever spent in my life. I wouldn't wish that amount of fear, anxiety or nausea on anyone. Not to mention the amount of white wine I consumed (just kidding – I was still pregnant after all!).

In that time, my husband and I learned to move forward with baby steps, trying desperately to maintain a reasonable amount of routine for our daughter, Bryn. She was, as children are, very much aware that something was terribly wrong. No matter how we comforted her, she noticed our moods, picked up on our wild emotions, and watched with curiosity as bouquet after bouquet of flowers arrived at our door.

She witnessed the hugs, the tears, the outbursts, and overheard, I am sure, more than one hushed phone call in which we explained what we knew so far to our concerned friends and family members. At last, we realized that we owed this little person the truth, at least in as much detail as her young mind could process. It was up to us, her parents, to do this right. No pressure.

We sat down with our beautiful, trusting, loving little girl and explained that we had something important to talk to her about. She was all ears and eyes (oh, those big, blue eyes would melt your heart).

I told her that mommy had a booboo, a cancer booboo, that the doctors needed to fix. I would go to the hospital where the doctors would take good care of me. They would take away my booboo and soon I would feel much better. We'd just have to play gently for a little while.

Did she understand? She nodded, wide eyed, and said in her 2-1/2 years-going-on-thirteen way, "I'm hungry. Get me a snack". And so I did. Our work here, at least for the moment, was done.

Chapter 11:
Meeting the Surgeon

What's a nice lady like you doing in a place like this?

The very morning after receiving my cancer diagnosis, Dr. MacGillivray was kind enough to meet with us at the hospital to discuss the details and answer our many questions.

She had encouraged me on the phone to bring as many people as I wanted to, so that between us, we would be able to fully take in the information she would share with us. We had all suffered a terrible shock, and she knew from her experience as a surgeon how hard this would be for my loved ones and me.

At 7:30 a.m., we piled into a small room in Ambulatory Care at the Guelph General Hospital to await The Breast Lady. With me were my husband, my sister and my dad.

It had been an unspoken understanding between us that Shelley would be the calm one, there to maintain consciousness if nothing else. Dad would be the note-taker, happy to keep his mind occupied with the details and cold hard facts. Jeff, God love him, would do his best to continue forming saliva in an already parched mouth, and I, the "cancer patient", would do whatever the hell I wanted to do, the details of which remained to be seen.

Even with my eyes closed tight, I found that I could still smell "it". You know "it," right? If you've ever been in a hospital, you understand what I'm referring to. The hospital smell. It's like a mix of bleach, bodily fluids and terror. Which I guess makes sense, given that terror may lead to bodily fluids, thus a need for bleach.

As it turns out, the smell of "it" got to me in record time. Shelley ran to get me a glass of water and Jeff lovingly rubbed my back, or was he just holding on for dear life? It was not going well.

I do recall Dr. MacGillivray, large Tim's coffee in hand, entering the room and instantly putting us all at ease with her genuine concern and patient, relaxed manner. She carefully explained that my particular type of breast cancer, invasive ductal carcinoma (it was weeks before I could remember that term) was considered to be "the garden variety type". The majority of breast cancers are this very kind. A small relief, I suppose, to have a form of breast cancer that, if nothing else, has been seen and treated a million times before. This is definitely one situation where it is better to be one of the crowd.

She also told me that she had, in fact, received the results of my needle biopsy *before* I had even been in to have my core biopsy. She had known then that it was cancer. As soon as she had received the positive results of my needle biopsy, she called the hospital to have me rushed in for my core biopsy to determine the extent of the cancer as much as possible. That would explain why, three times in a row, I had been called by people at Guelph General Hospital who were offering me new, earlier biopsy times, because they had had cancellations. I just thought at the time that for once my luck was good.

Get this: as soon as she saw my needle biopsy results, Dr. MacGillivray had called the hospital and held operating room time for me early in May, knowing that upon receipt of my core biopsy results, I would have to have a lumpectomy. Yes, a surgery date was tentatively set for me on May 4th. A note of this had been put in my hospital file. The same file that the core biopsy radiologist had referred to.

Suddenly, I had a flashback to my belly laugh with the core biopsy radiologist who had read the "wrong" file, the file that indicated I had already booked an operation of some kind in May. Hahaha. Less funny in hindsight. Then, eventually, very funny. Sometimes you just have to laugh.

At the end of our meeting with Dr. MacGillivray, I had given my consent to have a lumpectomy, a breast-conserving procedure in which the lump is removed as well as some tissue surrounding it. She would also remove the lymph nodes under my right arm. Both the breast tissue and lymph nodes would be examined under the microscope to provide greater details about the cancer and prognosis. We had a plan and were anxious to move forward.

Chapter 12:
My Deepest, Darkest Fears

Things that go bump in the night

Each night, as I awaited my surgery date, I would crawl into bed, pull the blankets tightly around me, and pray: "Please, God, don't let me die. Please, God, don't let me die. Please, God, don't let me die." On and on, sometimes for hours.

I had deep, dark visions of my family living without me. My father and sister. My husband with a new wife. My daughters, motherless. Bryn and a not-even-born-yet second daughter. We had already named her Dana.

I had been 20 years old and my sister 22 when our mom died of a brain aneurysm after about a month in the hospital. The hole in my heart and my life has never really gone away since my mother's death. To do that to my children was unbearable. Unthinkable. "Please God, don't let me die. I'm not done yet."

Chapter 13:
Finding the Second Lump

Calgon, take me away!

In the time between my diagnosis and surgery date, I was feeling the extreme pressure of living with cancer inside my body. I was terrified. I needed to find ways to help me relax, at least enough to sleep a little bit. No easy task.

Reading has always been one of my favourite ways to spend free time. There's nothing like a good Oprah pick at bedtime to help me slip into a new world, relax and, eventually, doze off with dreams of adventure, crisis, love and relationships. However, reading was not an option at this point, what with the hysteria and all. So, about halfway through my six-day marathon wait I opted for my next favourite thing in the world to do for relaxation - a long, hot bubble bath.

I tucked Bryn into bed and filled the tub with hot, near-burning, water (possibly a bad idea for a very pregnant woman, but desperate times call for desperate measures). Maybe the physical pain would numb the emotional pain, for a little while anyway. Let's just say lots and lots of bubbles were involved. And a glass of white wine (perhaps also not the best idea as a pregnant woman. We'll never speak of it again!).

I slipped into the boiling magic elixir, instantly feeling myself relax and breathe a little more slowly, more deeply. I fully immersed myself, only for a moment, and listened to the silence. Even the voices in my head were quiet for a change.

As I came up for air, I kept my eyes closed and rested my head on the sloped back of the tub. I just "was". I'm sure I passed several calm, wondrous minutes just "being" before I had the inexplicable urge to put my hand to my right breast. Bad idea.

As surely as I knew that two plus two equals four (and I was almost positive of that, although I admit that math has never been my strong suit), I knew that somehow, in some dark, mysterious way, a second cancerous lump had joined forces with the first.

The next morning, after a long, sleepless night in which I spent hours bargaining with God, I called Lisa, the receptionist at Dr. MacGillivray's office. I had spoken to Lisa on the phone a couple of times already, and, although we had not yet met, I knew I liked her. Sometimes you just know that someone "gets" you. She did. I asked her to have Dr. MacGillivray call me as soon as she possibly could. I had a problem. A large, hard, round one.

Thankfully, The Breast Lady knows the stress and anxiety related to all things cancer, and she was kind enough to return my call very quickly that same day. I explained to her that I had found a new lump very close to the original one. I was just this side of a complete nervous breakdown (OK, maybe just *that* side of one) and to be honest, I have no idea how she even understood a word that I said to her. I guess part of a surgeon's medical training must be a course on "Understanding the Language of Terror and Hysteria 101". I believe that my surgeon, thankfully, had graduated at the top of her class on that one.

She was amazing at calming me and putting my mind at ease, as much as humanly possible under the circumstances. Whatever it was, and it was very likely swelling from the core biopsy procedure, she would take a look before my surgery, and, if necessary, it would be removed along with any other bastard lumps (that last part I put in my words, not hers). Anything at all suspicious would be toast once she got in there. A good woman to have on my team, that's for sure.

Now I just had to get through the next few days before the surgery without any more surprises. My wise husband gave me the best advice ever at that particular time in my journey with breast cancer. He looked lovingly into my frightened eyes and said, "If you'd just stop feeling yourself up in the bathtub you wouldn't keep finding lumps." So wise. That's why I married him.

Chapter 14:
The Lumpectomy

Would you like one lump or two?

Three days after discovering the evil twin of lump number one, I found myself in the ever-creepy Guelph General Hospital, again. For the record, the hospital is actually clean, bright and warm, as far as hospitals go. But it's a hospital, so by definition it is creepy above all else.

My posse was with me: Jeff and Shelley, my mother- and father-in-law, Mary-Alice and Bob, and my sister-in-law, Erin, my dad and my step-mom, Dot. My peeps. I pity them, really. How did they manage to keep their retching hidden behind masks of calm?

Actually, most of them did. Jeff pretty much needed a room of his own to lie down in. As phobic as I am about all things hospital, Jeff may be the one person who fears them even more. Much more.

I was quickly led into a small partitioned cubicle equipped with a hospital bed, some technical gadgets and a curtain. I was given, yes, you guessed it, a charming gown, falling fashionably just below the knees (freshly shaven knees, I might add). Luckily, I was familiar with this style and had no trouble deciding that, once again, front opening was the way to go. I had really turned heads last time around. Besides, that look, in my opinion, will never get old.

I lay on the bed, pretending to be anywhere but there.

The nurse who had shown me to my cubicle returned to take my vitals and ask me some basic questions for my file. I felt comfortable enough at that time. As long as I was keeping busy and things were happening, I was okay. It appeared that we were going to stay on schedule, that my surgery would be underway at 1pm as planned.

There is definitely some comfort in keeping on schedule. It made me feel like everything was under control. Control of my environment was becoming increasingly important to my peace of mind at that stage in the process, given that, for all intents and purposes, I had lost control of what was happening inside my body.

As quickly as things had begun, so did they come to a screeching halt. I'm not sure why, but there was a long period of time between the nurse taking my information down and leaving, and my being greeted by a burly, awkward porter. Or maybe it just seemed like a really long time.

To pass the time (have you ever tried to pass time when time has actually stopped completely? It's even harder than it sounds), I made frequent trips to the bathroom, desperately clutching the front of my gown as I shuffled down the hall.

I was allowed one visitor in my "room" at a time, so my cheerleaders took turns keeping me company. Funny how none of us talked much about the impending doom, I mean, surgery. We found all manner of trivial topics to discuss, and stayed with the "think happy thoughts" concept, speaking with a slightly forced joviality. Everyone spoke of how *lucky* I was to have found the lump early and to have gotten OR time so quickly afterwards. What a blessing. I was feeling a lot of things as I waited for my name to be called, but *lucky* definitely wasn't one of them.

When the porter came in to wheel me to the operating room, I was filled with equal parts fear and relief. Fear of the unknown. Relief that soon the unknown would become "the known". I noticed nothing and no one as I travelled the halls by way of bed-on-wheels. I vaguely recall the sound of a voice whimpering obscenities. To this day, I hope it was the voice *inside* my head.

The porter parallel-parked me along the wall, by a window, in the hallway right outside the operating room. It's a surreal feeling to be lying there, so vulnerable, and listening to the voices of various medical staff. You know darn well that the voices are coming from inside *your* OR.

The voices are of people happily doing their jobs; sharing jokes, asking about each other's weekend plans, lining up the "instruments" (and hopefully setting the heavy drugs by your OR table for easy access). I realized as I lay there trembling (was it cold?) that people are in that very OR having surgeries every day. It was a first for me, but not for anyone else in the vicinity. It's a good thing that there are people who can do those hospital jobs. I never could.

The arrival of Dr. MacGillivray by my bedside calmed me immediately. Thank God she hadn't called in sick. She informed me that it wouldn't be much longer and asked if I had any questions. "What the f#$@!?" came to mind, but I held my tongue. Off she went to scrub up (or is it down?). My heart was thumping loudly, drowning out the voices in my head.

In the last minutes before my big "date", I noticed a familiar face watching me. It was my original OB/GYN, eyeing me and noticing my big belly protruding from beneath my heated blanket. He slowly approached my bedside in the hallway, and asked if I was pregnant. Yes.

He asked what I was doing there and I explained that I was having a lumpectomy. He looked surprised and then smiled. He quietly said, "Don't worry. It won't turn out to be anything. You're so young". If only he had known how badly I wanted to believe his words that day.

Finally, it was time. I was rolled into the operating room. I looked around. It was the first time I had ever been in an OR. I didn't know it at the time, but it would not be the last.

The room was bright, metallic and very cold. I'm not sure exactly why, but the moment I was helped from my rolling bed onto the metal table, I relaxed. This was it. At last. No more waiting. My number one priority was to get that cancer out of my body as quickly as possible. I knew I was in skilled, competent hands and I trusted Dr. MacGillivray completely. Now bring on the narcotics.

Just before the administration of my anesthetic, Dr. MacGillivray and her assistant propped me up partially on my right side with a sponge wedge. This was to keep me from lying perfectly flat on my back. At seven months pregnant, it was not healthy to lie flat with so much weight pressing down on me. For a moment I thought, "This is not very comfortable", and then I remembered that I would soon be going to my happy place, a place of comfort and deep, deep sleep.

Dr. MacGillivray asked me to open my gown. She said, "You thought that you felt something else in there somewhere. Show me where you feel it so I can check it out". My right hand instinctively touched the new lump and my surgeon reached over to feel for herself.

I will be blatantly honest here. I knew without the slightest doubt that there was a second, equally deadly, lump in my breast. No way was it swelling from the core biopsy. Thankfully, I had a surgeon who never brushed me off, who took me seriously and paid attention to my gut feelings.

I stared into her eyes without once blinking as her hand found mine. I slipped my hand away so that she could fully feel the hard mass that had so recently taken up residence next door to the first.

There was a time, maybe only a millisecond in length, when across the face of my surgeon I watched the unspoken words, "Holy S@$%!" appear. Her composure was regained so quickly that I wonder to this day if I really saw the flash of shock and disbelief that was so clear to me as I watched her closely for a sign. My gut feeling was hence confirmed.

Being a pro, Dr. MacGillivray regained her composure instantly, assuring me that yes, there definitely was another lump and that she intended to remove absolutely everything suspicious or unwanted from my breast while she was in there, including this new intruder.

Next, a gentle-natured woman introduced herself as my anesthetist. She explained how the process of putting me under would work and asked about allergies. Only seasonal. No ragweed in here, I was certain. Hook me up.

She began by inserting a small needle into a vein in my left wrist. She injected a sweet, heaven-sent miracle drug that truly made me drift off into slumber within moments. I recall the dimming of lights, the slowing of all action and the sudden quiet. At last, darkness.

Chapter 15:
My Recovery in the Hospital

Just say yes!

I awoke shaking. My teeth were chattering. It was very bright and very cold. I was told it was an effect of the anesthetic and it would wear off in time.

A few questions from the nurse, and I was being rolled back through the hallways from recovery to my room on the sixth floor. I was off to obstetrics so that the nurses and doctors could monitor not only my own, but also my unborn baby's well being.

I was brought to the back area of a large, multi-patient room. I was far enough in there that it almost felt like I was on my own. Or maybe it was the drugs. Either way, I was quite comfortable there. Jeff had come up with me and then my family followed soon after. They were relieved that the surgery was finally over.

I say that my surgery was "finally" over because it had not gone as smoothly as planned. In life, as we had begun to learn, there are many surprises.

Dr. MacGillivray explained to me, as she had already explained to my family in the waiting room while I slept, that when she went into my right breast to remove the original and second tumours (they had been 3-1/2 centimetres and 3.0 centimetres respectively, two centimetres apart), she had found a large area of what is called Ductal Carcinoma In Situ (DCIS).

DCIS is basically an area of pre-cancerous cells. So, she excised the DCIS away as well as removing both lumps. In addition to removing the tumours, she removed an area of tissue around them to have sent immediately to the lab. She wanted to determine whether or not she had clean, cancer-free margins before closing me up. She had successfully obtained clear margins around both tumours but was told there was still some DCIS to remove. She continued scraping until she was sure the margins were clear. When all was said and done, Dr. MacGillivray estimated that about a quarter of my right breast had been removed.

When she had received confirmation from the lab that all was clear, she had begun the second part of her assignment: the lymph node dissection. The lymph nodes under the arm, I had learned, were often the first place to which breast cancer would spread. By removing and examining these nodes taken from my armpit, it could be determined if the cancer had begun to spread outside the breast.

It was scary enough to fear breast cancer, but to fear breast cancer that had spread beyond the breast in search of other homes to settle in, was like a nightmare I couldn't wake up from. Or it would have been, had I not been as high as a kite and as happy as a clam. Drugs are good. Just say yes.

Speaking of drugs, I feel the need to remind you of my delicate condition. Poor baby Dana inside of me. It was so not about her! Yes, recall that I was approximately 7-1/2 months pregnant at the time of my lumpectomy. I remember my first pregnancy and how terrified I was after taking one regular-strength Tylenol to rid myself of a migraine that had gone on for two days. I had finally caved and taken the pill, worried sick that I had instantly done irreparable damage to my unborn child.

Fast-forward to pregnancy number two: here I lay, basking in the drugged-out stupour of a woman on heavy narcotics. Fetus or no fetus, I was in heaven.

I vaguely remember that night in the hospital, after all of my family members had gone home. I lay in my bed, right arm propped up with pillows to keep me comfortable. I found peace that night the likes of which I've never found since. Me - the one with the terror of all things medical. If I die, I remember thinking, everyone will be fine. Just fine. Great, even. If I live, everyone will be fine. Just fine. Great, even. I love my family so much. I love hospitals so much. I love surgeons so much. I love lumpectomies so much. Zzzzzzzzzzzzzzzzzz.

Sadly, a pregnant woman can only take so many drugs. With the morning came a sober, very different feeling. Pain. Bad pain. I was able to take some medication to control the pain, but nothing like what they'd given me throughout the night. My technicolour dreams had given way to a dark, black nightmare.

Dr. MacGillivray visited me that morning to see how I was feeling. She had filled out my release forms and asked me to let the nurses know when I felt ready to go home. Never, was my thought at that time. As much as I hated hospitals, I felt safe under the watchful eye of the nursing staff. To go home was a terrifying thought, one I hoped to put off for as long as possible.

Next visitor: Dr. Fraser. He sat on the edge of my bed and we talked briefly. He asked me when I was getting out of there, and I explained that I could go anytime, but would likely stay the week. Or month.

No, no, no. I needed to get home, away from all the "sick people", was how he put it. The sooner the better. "Pack your bag and get out of here." Damn him. I wanted to stay, but he made me question myself. I'll never admit to him that he was right about the going home idea. Never.

Chapter 16:
My Continued Recovery

My fairy stepmother

Late that afternoon, I did indeed decide to pack my bag and go home, to recover in the most beautiful room you've ever seen. That's where my step-mom, Dot, really comes into the picture.

All along, Dot had been a source of love and support to me. It was she who had urged me to "Let go, and let God". Not bad advice, even if it's easier said than done sometimes.

When Jeff helped me up the stairs to our guest room, the room we had decided would be my recovery room, I could not believe my eyes. I had recently bought a new, beautiful set of bedding, to brighten up my "sick bed", as I liked to call it ("*sick* bed" gets way more attention than "bed"). I had not had time to put the new bedding on the bed before my surgery. I guess I had run out of time, what with my busy schedule of feeling myself up, finding new breast lumps, worrying, dry heaving and shaking with fear.

As I entered the room, I was immediately surprised and overwhelmed with happiness. The bed was beautifully made, with the decorative pillows placed just so. Dot had also used her creative flair and sense of design to move furniture around, put calming pictures on the walls, and place some of my favourite knick-knacks on the dresser. The room looked exactly how I had pictured it in my mind, only better.

The best of all was that she had placed a plaque that I had bought for myself, only days before my lumpectomy, on the bedside table. It was facing the bed in such a way that I would be able to see it while sitting up in bed or lying down to rest. It said, "Trust in the Lord with all your heart and lean not on your own understanding. In all your ways acknowledge Him and He will make your paths straight" (Proverbs 3: 5-6). It gave me more peace and strength than anyone would believe.

I'm not sure if Dot knew it at the time, but her careful placement of that plaque did indeed remind me often to let go and let God.

Chapter 17:
Creating a Peaceful Recovery Space

Don't go away mad, just go away

In the early days of my recovery at home, Jeff and I had decided that it would be best for Bryn to go for some play time at nana Dot and papa Don's house in London. No need to terrify her with the physical realities of my illness. I figured that realistically I, too, would recover much better if I did not feel the need to put on a happy face for the sake of my toddler. A seeping drain sticking out of my side and a recovery from a major surgery without the help of anything more than the odd Tylenol 3 was not going to lend itself to happy faces, of that I was relatively certain.

Feeling guilty, as is the norm for most mothers at all times, I worried about sending my daughter away at such a difficult time. She had been through so much already. How would she cope without me? As I sat back and watched Bryn excitedly pack her own bag and head for the door, it dawned on me that the separation might indeed be harder on me than on my delicate flower.

What was I thinking? As if I could compete with nana and papa! Even the drain and the excitement of daddy working from home would pale in comparison to what they had to offer: chocolate for breakfast, monkeying around on the "jungle gym" (papa's treadmill), and getting away with absolutely every single thing that mommy and daddy had worked so hard to teach her *not* to do over the past 2-1/2 years! She kissed us goodbye before my surgery and was long gone, in her glory, before my return to my "sick bed".

Now I could focus on the disgusting reality that had become my life since the lumpectomy. If you think I was a sight to behold while finding the first lump back in the shower at 5 months pregnant, let me assure you at this stage of the game, I was in a category all of my own. The scars, the drain, the pale skin, the dark circles under my eyes, the unshaven everything (no woman in her final trimester of pregnancy can reach any parts that need to be shaved, let alone a pregnant woman in the amount of pain that I was experiencing). Yes, I was the poster child for bad luck.

Have you ever seen a drain coming out of someone's body? It's just not right. I'm not saying it didn't serve an important purpose (like allowing the vile fluids to exit my body in a neat and tidy fashion), but don't you think in this day and age there should be some other way? I guess for the average surgery patient, with enough Percocet, the whole drain business would be easily reduced to a foggy memory at best. Sans drugs, the drain was literally a thorn in my side for five long days.

In difficult times, not only do you learn to lean on your true friends when you need them, but you also get to take advantage of the people in your family, the poor bastards who didn't choose you but who feel a familial duty to help care for you. Lucky for me, my sister is not squeamish in the least. She can eat a bowl of spaghetti with meat sauce while watching "Trauma in the OR". Her strong stomach and experience with medical procedures (having become a veterinarian some years back) were *both* extremely helpful when it came time, morning and evening, to empty my drain. This task was simply not an option for me, given that I was physically unable to look at my drain, or myself, much less touch either. Not even with gloves. No way.

So I would shuffle up to my sister in the bathroom, struggle to get my camisole up and over my head with the least amount of pain (note to self: always wear button-down shirts while recovering from painful upper-body surgeries) and bare all, eyes tightly shut to the point of seeing stars. I would hear the squirting sound as the drain was emptied and wonder if death would really be that bad. Okay, I shouldn't even joke about that. Sorry God.

I'm guessing that it was at about this point in our "shared journey" with cancer that my husband seriously regretted not reading the fine print on our marriage certificate. It is, in fact, a legally binding document and yes, he is stuck with me for better *and* worse. Little did we know then, but my recovery from the lumpectomy was actually one of the "better" parts of our marital journey with cancer. The road ahead would be a winding one.

Chapter 18:
Mother's Day with Auntie Erin

Retail therapy

While recovering at home, Auntie Erin came to visit. Jeff and his sister have always had a great relationship. They are brother and sister, but would look like good friends to anyone watching them who didn't know better. They laugh and joke, tell it like it is, and, of course, have great taste in spouses.

At the time of this particular visit, Uncle Brian, Erin's hubby, was at home, in London, working. Erin had packed a bag and come to spend some time with Jeff, Bryn and me. It was at the height of pain and fear, and it would be an understatement to say that I was not myself. I was alternating between fits of rage, cursing the whole world for my bad luck, and episodes of curling up in the fetal position, crying uncontrollably. Good times.

Erin and I had the good fortune of having some time to talk, sister to sister, without interruption. She asked about how I was feeling and healing. Was I in much pain? I asked her if she was getting excited about the end of the school year, a summer away from the stress and chaos a primary teacher inevitably faces.

Soon, we moved out of our comfort zone and inched our way into the darker and never-before-mentioned topics of pain, suffering and even death. I remember us sitting together, talking intensely, crying and laughing. I told her about my fears, my terror of dying and leaving my children motherless. She asked me questions bravely, even when it must have made her literally tremble as she awaited my responses.

I also remember how strong she was. She kept it together for me more than I would have thought possible. Her feelings, fears and anxieties were clear, written all over her pale face, but never did she break down to the point that I found myself comforting her.

Yet, she is human and it was when we talked about my as-yet unscheduled chemotherapy and its known side effects that I watched her heart break. She excused herself to the bathroom and cried for a long while. I couldn't even imagine what she had to be feeling at that time. To watch a loved one suffer, to stand by and want so badly to make it all better, must be profoundly painful.

Interestingly, it was Mother's Day weekend. I was unable to think of anything but my daughter, Bryn, and her unborn baby sister, Dana. I wanted to celebrate Mother's Day like all of my friends. I wanted to experience that feeling of normalcy that I had always known until the diagnosis of cancer stole it away. I wanted to live. I wanted someone somewhere to promise me that I would get through this and live a long, healthy life. I wanted *my* mother.

Just one of many reasons I love Erin is that, after a bonding session that meant so much to me, a discussion that I believe brought us closer than we were before, she made a suggestion. The teacher in her, the planner, had a plan. Why didn't we go shopping for baby furniture, clothes and whatever else a newborn baby would need? Erin knew that little time and energy had been devoted to our baby-on-the-way due to the circumstances of the last weeks. An outing, a shopping spree, was just what we all needed to clear our heads and to find joy again. Some retail therapy was just what the doctor ordered.

We piled into the Ford Focus and headed downtown. Jeff and I had wanted a new baby dresser for the nursery. We decided to walk around the beautiful downtown area in search of the perfect furniture. Oddly enough, we had great luck almost immediately. A person's luck can't be that bad forever, right? It was inside the cluttered Goodwill store that we found "the one".

It was a beautiful white dresser with alphabet blocks as drawer knobs. How cute was that? And it would match the white crib perfectly. Sold! On our way out we also caved and decided to buy a gorgeous, hand-made wooden baby cradle. In our minds, this would be a doll toy for Bryn, not a real bed for Baby Dana.

Erin treated us to the dresser and we paid for the cradle and were once again heading out into the world. Funny, but life already looked a whole lot brighter. It was almost as if Erin had *known* about shopping therapy before that day.

The following morning was a Sunday, so we decided there was no reason not to go to church. We got dressed and cleaned up, and headed to the Lord's house. As we sat through the sermon, we were touched by the message. It was Mother's Day. It was a time to celebrate and remember our own mothers, as well as all of the women we knew who were mothers or caregivers of any kind.

It was a bittersweet day for me, missing my mom terribly and feeling the still raw fear that I might not live to mother my own girls for years to come. Erin, Jeff and I were all brought to tears throughout most of the service.

Since then, Erin and I have talked about what the people around us must have thought. Indeed, they may have wondered what sadness and pain we were experiencing. Who knows what hidden pains of their own they were experiencing that day? We all hold our suffering up to God at church, praying for the strength to endure it, one day at a time.

I still look back on that visit and am thankful for Erin. She knew we needed her, and better yet, she knew we needed to get out and take our minds off the cancer, the pain and the worry. We needed a teacher, a prayer partner and a sister. In Erin, we got them all.

Chapter 19:
The Pathology Report

A perfect score!

As difficult as the early days of recovery were, I can say that we were all relieved to have the lumpectomy behind us. Still, we could only relax so much. We were anxiously awaiting one more very important call. We had been told that it would not take long to receive the results of the pathology report. We wondered what the report would say. Had my cancer spread to the lymph nodes? How much damage had been done inside my body? Was there more bad news to come?

I'm a firm believer that things happen for a reason. For example, I think it was Dr. Fraser who gave us this particular news because we needed to hear it from him. We had grown to trust him and feel comfortable around him. He was an integral part of our team.

Dr. Fraser himself led Jeff and me to his tiny, cluttered office. You know, it looked exactly the way I pictured his office would look. Stacks of papers, books, folders. Stuff everywhere. I'm sure his "filing system" works for him. He's never lost my file, so it can't be *that* bad.

We were really only there for a regular check-up, to make sure that the pregnancy was rolling along smoothly. Little did we know that Dr. Fraser had received a copy of the pathology report and he was looking forward to sharing the good news.

He opened my file, took a look for a moment and smiled that Doc Fraser smile. He said that all of my lymph nodes were clear. Cancer-free. All 15 out of 15. Not that I'm saying marks matter, but come on, that's a *perfect* score! If ever there was a time for me to ace a test, this was it! Complete relief for the first time in a long, long time. Phew. Thanks Dr. Fraser.

Chapter 20:
The Consultation at Juravinski Cancer Centre

Becoming a Team Player

After having had time to recover somewhat from my surgery, I received a phone call from a receptionist at the Juravinski Cancer Centre in Hamilton, Ontario. She had an appointment booked for me with Dr. Richard Tozer, the man who would be my medical oncologist from that point forward. I was anxious to meet him and discuss the "What next?" question that had been on my mind since the surgery was completed.

Before the day of my big appointment, I had called for my family to support me. Jeff and I had arranged for Grandpa Bob to stay at our house and entertain Bryn (Bob is clearly where Jeff gets his fear of hospitals and there was no way we'd force him to come along to this appointment). My dad would drive Shelley and me to the meeting. Jeff and his mom would travel together, meeting us there. Again, I had been encouraged to bring as many people as possible to this appointment because it would be long and full of difficult information to hear and retain.

As we drove in silence, I could feel the bile rising in my throat. My whole life I had been terrified of cancer. I don't know if it was because our family had been so riddled with it over the years, or if it was simply an unknown, scary thing that I associated automatically with an early, painful, ugly death.

In any case, this was certainly a situation in which I was forced to face my worst fear. Head on. It seemed a dramatic way to go about it. I would have much preferred to go on the Dr. Phil show and have him expose me somehow to my fears without them hitting quite this close to home.

We parked and walked up to the building, passing many bald people - men and women of all ages. I looked away. I am ashamed to this day that I was unable at that time to smile and say hello to the people passing by. They represented my worst fear and I was not ready to see them as everyday regular people, as I was. Somehow, they had to be different from me. I could *not* be like them.

We entered Juravinski and followed the signs to Clinic D, the waiting area for Dr. Tozer's patients. I handed in my health card, introduced myself as Marcie *Adams* (I really should change my name on my health card), and we took our seats in the waiting lounge.

Again, I looked everywhere but up. The carpets at Juravinski Cancer Centre are lovely, very clean and well kept. Also, did you know that many people in a cancer centre waiting room have beautifully pedicured toenails? It's true, in my experience. Yes, those are the things I noticed. I did not see anyone's face. I did not once make eye contact. This was *not* happening to me.

To be completely honest, I admit that I did sneak peeks around me from time to time, often enough to notice that, as far as cancer centres went, this one was beautiful. It's hard to imagine such a centre as being beautiful, but it really was. Surprisingly, it was bright, nicely decorated, full of colour and not at all what I had conjured up in my terrified mind. The prison-like surroundings of my imagination were quickly, and quite easily, replaced by a welcoming, friendly reality. Cool. Too bad about the sick people.

When my name was called, I darted for the nurse who asked me to step onto a massive walk-in scale. It certainly wasn't like any other scale I'd seen before. I wondered if it was common practice for elephants to be treated at cancer centres. Later it dawned on me that it was designed to accomodate people in wheelchairs. At the time I just thought it was cruel and unnecessary to emphasize the weigh-in process. However, my weight was recorded (something all pregnant women are used to, whether they like it or not) and we were directed to yet another room, the consultation room. There were two seats and five people. I sat down automatically. It was really all about me, after all. The rest could fight it out for all I cared.

In walked a very brightly dressed, beautiful woman with the best eyes and smile you could ever hope to see when at a cancer centre. She introduced herself as nurse Judy and shook our sweaty, shaking hands. My people introduced themselves and we were ready to move forward, whatever that would entail.

Judy began by explaining to us the specifics related to "my" cancer. She told us my cancer was called Invasive Ductal Carcinoma. My tumours had been estrogen- and progesterone-receptor negative, meaning they did not "feed on" my body's own hormones. Not those hormones, anyway. My cancer was "multi-focal", simply meaning it was found in more than one spot in the breast. Best of all, it was gone. My tumours and DCIS had been successfully removed by means of a lumpectomy. As Judy put it, the cancer didn't "live there" anymore.

Next, I answered a series of personal questions, in front of my entire family. I have always considered my family to be quite close-knit (with a few exceptions during my tempestuous teen and early adult years, but we won't go into that), but did they really need to know when I began menstruating and for how long I had been on birth control pills? Too much information for everyone, I'm sure. Judy wrote down the answers to my questions and made me feel as comfortable as possible under the circumstances. I had just met her but was already so glad to have her on my team.

After taking my personal and medical histories, Judy introduced us to Dr. Alcivear, or "Big Al", as we were asked to call him. He was, as his nickname would suggest, a very tall man. He was warm, charming, professional and very caring. He had a big personality to match his size. Big Al was a resident working with Dr. Tozer. He spoke to me a bit more about the specifics of my cancer diagnosis and the treatment plan we were about to undertake. Then, Big Al, with his big hands, proceeded to do a physical exam of my very tender, recently lumpectomied right breast. Of course, he was extremely conscious of my state of continuing recovery and did what he could to keep the pain to a minimum. He was gentle but certainly made sure that everything felt right; no worrisome lumps, bumps or bogey men in that breast since the surgery. As hard as he tried to conduct a pain-free exam, it was quite some time before I could look back on that experience and laugh.

One thing in particular stands out in my mind when I think of my meeting with Big Al. I recall him explaining to me how chemotherapy worked and I was obviously terrified at the mention of the word. He looked directly at me with his big, brown eyes and said, "You can do this". He meant it. At that stage in my life, I still needed someone else to believe that, and it felt good to hear him say it. We spoke about Big Al on the drive home that day and my entire family had had the same first impression of him. He was another keeper for my team of medical practitioners.

Last, but certainly not least, in walked my cancer care team captain, medical oncologist extraordinaire, Dr. Richard Tozer. He entered the room, introductions were exchanged and, from that moment on, I have trusted him to the point that if he told me to jump off a cliff, I would seriously look into the purchase of a parachute. That kind of trust is necessary when dealing with the life and death issues of cancer treatment. I'm pretty sure Dr. Tozer has other patients, too, but I like to think of him as all *mine*.

All joking aside, Dr. Tozer is not only very bright, experienced and talented in all things related to cancer treatment, but he is able to talk to people. This, I tell you, is a good thing. We spent a lot of time with him, and it helped immensely that he made us feel comfortable, that he spoke in a way that was clear but not condescending and, of course, we were almost positive that he knew what he was talking about.

When all of the introductions had been made, Dr. Tozer got down to the business of explaining in detail what my treatment plan would be. I had been prepared for the fact that chemotherapy and radiation were likely possibilities, but this was the day to find out for sure.

Yes, he assured me, chemotherapy was necessary. Based on my young age and family history, as well as the stage and grade of the tumours, this was the most aggressive form of treatment available. Technically the cancer was gone, so chemotherapy was a preventative measure. At that point, I was all for aggression when it came to kicking cancer's butt. Radiation was likely to follow chemotherapy, but at that point, the focus was on chemically treating any cancer cells that might be lingering in my body, unwanted and undetected.

The type of chemotherapy that I would be treated with was called A.C.T. Each letter stands for a long drug name. The A is for Adriamycin, often referred to as the Red Devil because of its bright red colour and often brutal side effects. The C is for Cyclophosphamide and the T is for Taxol. Dr. Tozer told us that I would be receiving eight chemotherapy treatments in total. The first four treatments would consist of both Adriamycin and Cyclophosphamide. The final four treatments would consist of Taxol on its own.

My chemo schedule would be every three weeks for approximately six months. A long time to be bald and sick, I remember thinking as he spoke. The fact that I would have a newborn baby to care for was a reality that I had basically learned to push to the back corners of my mind. For now, I would learn all that I could about my chemotherapy regimen and deal with the rest as it happened.

The plan was for me to begin chemotherapy after delivering my baby on her natural due date. From a medical perspective, there was no reason to deliver Dana early. By the time I had fully recovered from the lumpectomy, it would be very close to my due date anyway. Dr. Tozer assured me that the timing worked out well. I was due to have my baby right around the time that he wanted me to begin my chemotherapy. How convenient.

So, we would go home and I would await labour, praying to God that my fear of starting chemotherapy would not overshadow the excitement of the birth of my second daughter. Already, she had been through so much.

Chapter 21:
The Birth Plan

I wanna be sedated...

I drove back to Dr. Fraser's office with lots on my mind. I had been to Hamilton to meet my cancer-care team. I had a plan. Now, one small detail remained: The birth. Right, I was having a baby soon and had spent very little time thinking about life with a newborn. Cancer has a nasty way of taking over your life, if you're not careful.

I handed in my health card, sat in the waiting room and looked around. Lots of tired, uncomfortable-looking women, all of whom were probably praying that they would have their baby *soon*. Just get it out. Yes, I believe that's why a pregnancy is so long. You have nine months to get used to the idea of a baby. You also have nine months to become so uncomfortable with the baby on the *inside* that the idea of getting the baby *out* is far less frightening than the idea of the baby staying *inside* forever!

When my name was called, I followed the nurse to be weighed and felt much more comfortable on the human-sized scale than the uber-scale at the cancer centre. Inside the small patient waiting room, the nurse took my blood pressure and tested my urine. Luckily, I had given up steroids so was relatively certain I'd pass that test. Haha.

Dr. Fraser knocked lightly and came right in. I was always happy to see him. I filled him in on the latest news, Dr. Tozer's plan to begin chemotherapy after I had my baby whenever she decided to come naturally. He was pleased to hear that there was no medical need to induce Dana too soon, and that it was within our control to deal with the birthing as we saw fit. That's where things got interesting.

Since my lumpectomy, I had been in a great deal of pain on a regular basis. It was still extremely difficult to wear a seatbelt when driving. It hurt to walk up and down stairs. It hurt to lie on either side to sleep. It hurt to do pretty much everything. There were many times when I was brought to tears from the pain, the constant, never-ending-reminder-of-breast-cancer pain.

At this particular appointment, since we were talking about the birth plan, I reminded Doc Fraser of the hideous breast pain, the cancer, the difficulty eating, the cancer, the varicose veins, the cancer, the heartburn, the acid reflux and the cancer. Did I mention the *cancer*? As it turned out, I was due for a mental breakdown and he was about to witness it. Poor bastard.

I told him that I had thought a lot about it and had come to a decision. I was going to have the baby by a planned Cesarean section. I was too tired, too sore and too weak to push a baby out of my body. I just couldn't do it. The thought of giving birth made me want to vomit. It was simply not an option for me. I wanted to be knocked out, possibly unconscious, and for him to just take the baby out and, if possible, raise it for a few months since things were going to be pretty hectic, what with the cancer and all. That was my plan. So, let's get our calendars out and pick a birth date for Dana, Doc. How is June 15th for you?

I am guessing that I am not the first completely hysterical pregnant woman that Dr. Fraser has ever had to deal with. The guy's an obstetrician; it's kind of his job, right? He listened patiently while I ranted and cried and felt sorry for myself. He smiled and nodded. He assured me that it was all going to be within my control. "If, when the big day comes, you say to me you want a Cesarean section, then a Cesarean section you will have. I can't promise you that I won't try one more time to convince you to go the natural route, but you *will* have the delivery you choose."

There was, he explained simply, a great deal to be said for not having to recover from another major surgery, after all that my body had been through already. A C-section would certainly take more out of me in the long run than a natural birth. Dr. Fraser also wondered out loud if my recovery from a Cesarean section would postpone my chemotherapy. We definitely didn't want that to happen.

Finally, he asked me to give some thought to the following idea: was it possible that, for me, giving birth naturally– the act of physically using my body's wisdom and strength to deliver my child into the world– would be empowering? Maybe I would come out of such an experience feeling stronger and better about my body. He suggested, as I glamorously wiped my nose on my sleeve and waddled to the exit sign, that I wait a while before making a final decision about the birth. It was fine with him, if, when all was said and done, I decided that a Cesarean section was what I really wanted. But we had some time left yet before a decision was necessary.

I've told you about this man before. He's good. Really good. "Just think about it," he said. "We'll talk again soon. It will all be your decision when the time comes." Damn him.

Chapter 22:
It's a Girl!

You had me at epidural

You will not be surprised to learn that, when the time came to make a decision, I went ahead and gave Dr. Fraser the OK to book me for an induction, two weeks early, and it would be natural. I use the term "natural" very loosely. There would be drugs. Lots and lots of narcotics, the likes of which you can only buy on the black market (in the shady parts of big cities). No way was I playing the hero this time.

Thank God Doc threw me a bone. For purely compassionate reasons he recommended the induction of Dana two weeks before my actual due date. He felt that I had waited long enough, been through enough and that, hell, it was time to celebrate something really really good in my life. A welcome event for all involved. Or maybe he just wanted to do it before my next meltdown?

This would also give me three weeks with my baby at home before I was set to begin chemotherapy treatments, a reality that loomed on my mind at all times, at least on some level. In any case, Dana was scheduled to arrive sometime on June 29th, 2005. I absolutely could *not* wait!

On the morning of June 29th, Jeff and I arrived at the Guelph General Hospital at 8 a.m. on the dot. Bags in hand. Stomachs in mouths. We made our way up to the sixth floor: Obstetrics.

We were greeted by a friendly nurse who handed me some paperwork to fill out. I should have filled it out much more slowly. Once it was handed in, there was a long, long wait. It's hard to come up with things to talk about while you await induction of your baby. The weather outside or the headlines in the newspaper didn't really seem terribly pertinent at that moment. So we sat, in silence, each of us trying not to breathe. Breathing, of course, would force us to smell "it" and smelling "it" would undoubtedly end in at least one pool of vomit. So we held our breath and prayed for Dr. Fraser to get the show on the road.

By 9 a.m. I was settled in my own room. I had on my usual hospital get-up and was stretched out and anxious for the next step. Doc determined that the best way to begin was simply to break my water and let me walk around the floor for an hour or so, to see if that was enough to get labour started naturally. Sounded like a good plan to us.

The breaking of my water was quick and painless, just how I like those sorts of things to be. Dr. Fraser did the perfect break. Even *he* was proud of his work! He said he'd never had such a textbook flood as that. Is that too much information? With that done, I was led to the hallway to walk until something happened "down there".

I have mentioned my husband's discomfort with hospital settings. I should probably also mention that, unbeknownst to me, before arriving at the hospital that morning, Jeff had taken not one, but *two* Gravol pills to keep his nausea at bay. He had anticipated that the whole hospital experience would be really ugly, and was being pro-active. It figures he would choose *this* time of all times to plan ahead.

The area of hallway that we were walking in was a big L shape. We simply went up and down the L over and over again. This was great the first few times. We were chatting away, joking even. Good times. By about the fourth or fifth lap, I began to notice that I was ahead of Jeff.

At one point, I was talking to him and didn't hear a response. I turned to look for him, and he was back at the last window. He was half standing, half sitting, head in hands, in the middle of the hallway. As funny as it is looking back, at the time, let me assure you, I was *not* laughing.

I waddled back to my hopeless husband and asked him politely what the hell his problem was. Who was the one with the full-sized newborn on the inside of her body refusing to come out? Who was the one who hadn't slept in God-only-knows how many months? And whose fault was it that I was in this condition anyway?

As a husband, I have to tell you that Jeff is fantastic. I wouldn't trade him for anyone else. As a birthing coach, however, I probably should have shopped around a bit.

He ended up going back to my room to sleep it off while I walked the halls alone. Cursing him. Plotting against him. Planning my new life without him as soon as this baby was out in the world. Needless to say, I was really glad I had let him talk me into keeping this birth experience for only the two of us. He had insisted that no one else be there at the hospital with us. It was our last baby. Our last chance to experience this wondrous event as a couple. Just the two of us. Bastard.

An hour of walking came and went without any signs of Wee Nolan wanting to make contact with the outside world. I shuffled back to Jeff's room and asked if he would scooch over so I could lie down and rest my aching body on "his" hospital bed while we waited for Dr. Fraser to return. He moved. Good choice.

It wasn't long before the doctor was back, ready to check for "progress". Nope. The walking hadn't done the trick. Plan B was to begin a Petocin drip, a drug to bring on labour in all its fury. This plan would allow me to spend some magical quality time with my birthing coach, so I agreed to go along with it. I woke up Jeff to tell him the great news. Things were really going to start happening now. He was thrilled (and by "thrilled" I mean "semi-conscious").

Dr. Fraser left to put the order in for my Petocin, and while I waited a young, kind man walked in and introduced himself as Dr. "Sent-From-Heaven", the anesthetist. OK, I can't remember his exact name, so I've made one up for the purpose of this story. Dr. S-F-H explained that he had talked to Dr. MacGillivray earlier that morning and she had told him all about me. Dr. Fraser had kept her in the loop about my progress, pregnancy and due date. My sweet anesthetist was well aware of my difficult experience over the last few months and wanted me to know that he would ensure that I had no more pain. I believe I told him that I loved him.

I had two options for pain relief. Drugs now or drugs later. They were the only two options that had ever come into consideration around the whole birth idea. I opted for the "drugs now" plan and Dr. S-F-H was off to prepare for my epidural.

I must say that the experience of an epidural, a needle in the spine that will numb a person from the waist down, was somewhat different the second time around. By the time I was given my epidural when I was in labour with Bryn, I had already been experiencing severe labour pains for quite some time. At that point, a large needle in each eye would have sounded great if I knew it would stop the pain. This time, I had not even started having contractions, or at least none that I could feel. As such, the idea of a large needle in my spine was slightly less appealing.

I sat on the edge of my bed, gown open to the back for a change, and held a pillow around my belly. My husband had started coming out of his Gravol-induced stupor by this time and was there, wobbling by my side, not making eye contact with anyone as far as I could tell. Just having him there gave me great strength (an angry woman is a strong woman, you know).

The anesthetist spoke gently and calmly to me, explained what he was going to do before doing it and made sure I was OK. He even said that he would make sure my breast pain didn't bother me while I was in labour. At that point a moment without any breast pain was inconceivable to me. It had been so long since I had lived without pain. In my opinion, anesthetists don't get nearly enough credit.

The psychological side of getting a needle in your spine is probably the worst part, as with so many things. I had no labour pains to distract me or make me desperate for relief. I felt just like always. I was fine. Yet, I was about to get an epidural to relieve pain that I wasn't even having yet. Now *that* is good service.

In went the needle. I felt the cool rush. I breathed deeply. Jeff stopped breathing entirely, but only temporarily. And we were done. Personally, I would recommend this procedure to any woman who finds herself with a baby inside of her that has to come out.

I thanked Dr. Sent-From-Heaven, who then moved on to make someone else's life better. In came Dr. Fraser with the Petocin. A nurse, Norma, hooked me up to an IV drip and Doc gave orders to start the Petocin off very slowly and to wait and see what happened. Sometimes it doesn't take much to get the body into labour.

We waited. Waited. Waited. Jeff dozed off with a newspaper on his lap, stretched out on the cot under the window. I was anxious and excited. I finished my book. Thank God for Oprah's book club. I had packed a novel at the last minute, chuckling to myself at the thought of having the time or energy to read it while in the hospital.

I could no longer feel my lower half, nor my right breast. Now how in the world did that darling anesthetist get the freezing to go straight to my breast? I want that man to get an award of some kind. The Nobel Peace Prize, maybe? I actually just enjoyed a pain-free existence for a while, listening to the nurses out at their station.

I wondered about my unborn daughter. Who was this little angel that God had blessed me with? I was acutely aware of the fact that, had I found the breast lump only a few months sooner, there was no way I (we) would have decided to have a second child. We would have been thankful for our one beautiful, perfect daughter and left it at that. It was clear to me that this infant was meant to be.

I considered the name we had chosen for our second, miracle baby. Dana Nancy Nolan. Nancy after my mom. Dana because Jeff and I had stumbled on it early on in the "name-game" and couldn't get past it. We loved it immediately and felt it was "the name".

I thought about it and its meaning, which is "Danish", or "from Denmark". Very romantic, don't you think? Clearly we chose the name because we loved the sound of it, not because the meaning was close to our hearts. I wish that her name meant something like "Brave Angel" or "Miracle of God" or even "Precious Gem". No such luck. And yet, I knew in my deepest heart and soul that it was Dana Nancy inside of me. I couldn't wait to meet her.

Most of the day went by uneventfully. It seemed wrong to ask to have our room television hooked up, but believe me, it crossed our minds. As with so many happily married couples, we had long since run out of things to talk about and just wanted to find a movie we could agree on. Not a great "birthday story" for Dana's baby book, though, so we just waited in comfortable, loving silence.

At one point, as I lay awake, looking around my room and trying to overhear what the nurses were all laughing about at their station, I received a visitor. The Breast Lady, Dr. MacGillivray, poked her head in to see how I was doing. She told me that Doc Fraser had kept her informed of my progress and had let her know that I was being induced that day. She had wanted to wish me luck before "the action" began.

As it turned out, Doc MacGillivray wanted to be long gone before I actually went into strong, active labour. Too funny that a general surgeon would get woozy at the thought of labour and delivery! She was fine with removing body parts from living people, but childbirth was just too much to stomach! That pretty well proved my theory that there is nothing remotely *natural* about delivering a baby. It's just not right. Even my surgeon agrees. But I digress.

Time seemed to go on endlessly until, seemingly all of a sudden, my contractions went from mild and sporadic to intense and regular. They were strong and close together, and we had a delivery on our hands! My epidural had worn off just enough that I was still relatively comfortable but could feel the pressure of the contractions and knew instinctively when I needed to start pushing. The nurses told me that the pushing stage would likely last a while, so I might as well get started and once the baby got closer they would call for Dr. Fraser.

I did what they always tell you to do. I closed my eyes, put chin to chest and gave a mighty push "from my bottom". Next, I heard the nurses hollering, "Stop! Stop! Don't push anymore! The head is coming!" and then someone bolted to get Doc

Fraser and I remained very still, holding mid-push and waited for further instructions. Let's just say that when my first daughter was born, she literally came tearing into the world. I did *not* want a repeat performance of that. So when they said to stop pushing, I sure did.

Dr. Fraser did not let me down. He was there in record time, ready to bring my baby into the world, and, more importantly, into my arms. He did whatever it is he needed to do "down there" (sometimes less information is more) and coached me calmly to give a slow, calculated push. As my bald little beauty's head emerged, Doc urged me to feel her soft, warm head. I believe he had to say it two or three times before I registered what was happening.

I reached down and felt the most amazing thing I believe I will ever feel as long as I live. My daughter, Dana Nancy, left my body and joined my life forever. It was so sudden. So amazing. Straight from my womb to my heart. Instantly. As quickly as she was in the world, Doc had her in my arms, all warm, sticky, cheesy seven pounds and one ounce of her. Perfect. Perfect. Perfect. Jeff and I had, for the second time in the history of the world, created a perfect human being. We ruled.

And then my daughter cried. In the tradition of small bundles of Adams/Nolan fury, Dana was a livewire. Mommy's little girl, all right!

Chapter 23:
The Abdominal Ultrasound

I don't know if I can stomach this

Only a week after Dana's arrival, I found myself at the Henderson Hospital in Hamilton. Jeff was with me. I was scheduled to have an abdominal ultrasound, to make sure that there was no cancer in my liver.

As if an abdominal ultrasound isn't horrifying enough, the hospital we were walking through was dark, old and not unlike something you'd see in a horror movie. How romantic; it was our first date since we had had Dana. We held hands (I'd like to say it was out of love, but admit that it had a lot more to do with each of us keeping the other from running away).

After signing in, we were told to wait in a little waiting area until they were ready for me. Again, good luck making small talk in this particular situation. We had long ago given up even trying. We looked around, absent-mindedly flipped through very old copies of Reader's Digest and were lost in our own thoughts. I can't speak for Jeff, but my thoughts at that time cannot be printed here. We'll leave it at that.

I believe we both jumped up when my name was called. A lady led us into a small, dark room and asked me to put on a little gown and strip down to my underwear. On a different kind of date, alone without our kids, Jeff might have been thrilled to find my clothes in a heap on the floor. Not here, however. No, he was working hard just to remain conscious at that moment.

I put on my blue gown, admired myself briefly and hopped up on the bed. I sat, perfectly shaven legs dangling over the side, and looked at my husband. He was slouched in a little chair looking terrified. God, what was he thinking as he sat there? He must have wondered how his life had taken such a nasty turn. He was a good man. A great man, in fact. A loving husband. The best father around. And yet, here he sat in a dark room awaiting his wife's next test. He didn't deserve any of it. None of us did.

When the ultrasound technician entered the room and introduced herself, we liked her instantly. She was very friendly, calm and easy to talk to. She explained what she was doing as she did it and answered my questions simply. I was lying in such a way that I could see part of the screen. I was not familiar with what a healthy liver looked like, so trying to assess how it was going based on what I saw was tricky.

As far as I can tell, unless you're trained to read those things, all ultrasound images make it look as though there are massive areas of disease everywhere. I soon opted for the "looking around the room" approach. Much more relaxing.

Not more than half an hour or so later, the procedure was done and I was free to change back into my clothes. The technician told us she'd give me a minute to get dressed and would be back. I got myself ready, sat with Jeff and we waited. We knew that this woman would not likely tell us what she saw. We'd have to wait for someone to call us with the results. Still, we were scared.

At last the technician returned (probably three minutes later, but to us it was an eternity). She told us that she knew it was Friday and that we'd be worried all weekend long, wondering and waiting. She said she wanted us to know right then and there that everything looked great; she saw absolutely no sign whatsoever of any disease. I had a perfectly healthy liver. Have a good weekend. Oh yes, we sure would!

We thanked her profusely and may have told her she was our new best friend in the world. Then we got the hell out of there.

Chapter 24:
The Bone Scan

Throw me a bone!

I have already mentioned several times my dislike for medical situations, so it should seem obvious by now that any procedure with the words "bone" or "scan" in it was going to be a problem for me. Big time.

We had all known since the meeting with my medical oncologist, Dr. Tozer, that I was being scheduled for this test. It was, of course, necessary to make sure that there was no sign of cancer in my bones. It was a routine procedure for anyone who would be undergoing cancer treatments. The bone scan was booked for shortly after Dana's birth.

This is where I say, "Thank God for female friends". All the medical tests were taking their toll on me and I was a basket case. A husband is a great thing to have and mine is definitely the best you'll find, but sometimes you just need to talk to a woman about things.

Tanya and I go way back. I lived in Halifax, Nova Scotia, from the end of Grade 4 until the end of Grade 6. My dad had accepted a work transfer there, knowing it would only be for a short time, so our family could experience life in the Maritimes. I've always believed that things happen for a reason. I believe my family moved there so that Tanya and I could meet. My life would never have been complete without her in it.

Tanya and I became inseparable from the first moment we met. It has been more than 20 years now and our friendship is stronger than ever. We have grown up together, albeit by long-distance, and have been in each others' weddings, celebrated the births of four gorgeous children between us and have spent about a billion hours talking about a diverse range of issues, from the profound to the downright ridiculous. Since the majority of those hours have been spent on the phone, we feel we are in large part responsible for Bell Canada's success.

I should mention that Tanya is a nurse. She has the ideal personality and temperament for it, too. She is fun, easy-going, compassionate, empathetic and strong. She was the obvious person for me to turn to when the fear of my bone scan started keeping me up at night. I couldn't breathe when I thought about it. I knew from experience that she would say the perfect thing, whatever that was, to put my mind at ease and give me the courage to face this next test.

Tanya has a long history of saying the perfect thing, but this time she said the *most* perfect thing to date. She said, "I've booked a flight and will be arriving the day before your bone scan. I'm staying for four days. I'll be right beside you all the way." And then she was here. In person. Now *that* is friendship.

On bone scan day, we walked up to the receptionist at the Guelph Imaging Centre and handed in my health card. We sat and tried not to laugh hysterically. We had to actually avoid making eye contact to stay composed. It didn't seem like the right place for fits of laughter. Nerves have a strange way of manifesting themselves, usually inappropriately where Tanya and I are concerned. This was no exception.

A nurse called us in and led us to a large, bright open room. It was divided into sections. She explained that she would be injecting me with radioactive dye. It would take a few hours for it to get through my system, so we would be able to leave and return later for the actual bone scan. I was all for leaving. It was the returning part I didn't care for.

We drove to Tim Hortons and had a large half and half. If you've never tried this, I strongly recommend it. It was Tanya who first introduced me to it years ago and it has been my favourite comfort drink ever since. Well, that and wine.

Anyway, it is half coffee and half French vanilla cappuccino. I find the cappuccino too sweet on its own, but the combination of it with Tim's coffee is amazing. It really doesn't take much to make me happy.

So we drank and talked, keeping an eye on the time. We'd never had trouble passing hours together before, but this time was different. We were both anxious and preoccupied. We'd feel so much better when the test was complete.

Exactly three hours later, we walked up to the receptionist to let her know we were back. A nurse came and took me right away. No more waiting. I was asked to lie down on a bed, fully clothed (but I had shaved my legs for this!). The nurse briefly read over my file and must have misunderstood the pregnancy part. She asked me when my baby was due. "She's 2-1/2 weeks old," I replied. Gee, I guess I hadn't lost much baby weight yet. Again, no eye contact with Tanya. It was a bone scan. No laughing. No laughing. No laughing.

The machine was programmed and I was told to lie still. I could talk and even turn my head to face Tanya, except while the scanner was over my head. This procedure would take 60 minutes. Starting now.

It took very little time before we fell into our old standby routine: Food talk. We are food people, Tanya and I. We love to eat and don't care who knows it. To pass the hour, Tanya began to tell me about a little family-owned Greek restaurant that she and her husband, Mike, and their two beautiful children, Megan and Jacob, had gone to recently.

I remember her describing in great detail the several different courses. The smells, the colours, the tastes. The huge portions. It sounded amazing. Souvlaki, spanokopita, hummus, tsatsiki sauce, lamb, Greek salad, rice, big roasted potatoes, and baklava to die for.

For nearly an hour, I was taken away to a little Ma and Pa restaurant in Halifax. I was not on a hard bed getting a bone scan. How does Tanya always know just what to say to make things better?

Chapter 25:
Preparation for our Teaching Day with Nurse Judy

Whine and cheese

While Tanya was in town for my bone scan, it just so happened that I had another important appointment to attend. It was one that I was happy to have her join me for.

My oncology nurse, Judy, at the Juravinski Cancer Centre, had set up an appointment for what she called a "teaching day". It was a meeting at which we would have the opportunity to really talk about my upcoming chemotherapy treatments. She would tell me all about it and answer my many questions so that I felt more prepared and comfortable when I went for my first treatment. I should mention that this is a service only offered by Judy to Dr. Tozer's patients and I am so thankful that she went the extra mile to put my mind at ease.

The night before my teaching day, Tanya and I decided we should read the information pages I had been given about my chemotherapy. I had a printout for each of the three drugs I would be receiving. We felt we needed to prepare ourselves fully for the meeting with Judy and figured that reading about it might help us formulate our questions. I had yet to really read any of it on my own, what with the terror and all. Chemotherapy. Shiver.

Tanya went into the kitchen to get us a snack while I rooted around for the info sheets. I found them, set them on the coffee table and got out the wine. She got out the wine glasses. The big ones were easier to reach in the cupboard than the small ones, so she went with the big ones. Good call. We'd only have half a glass anyway. We needed clear heads for the task at hand.

The "snack" that Tanya had decided on was basically a brick of cream cheese rolled in dill, wrapped in Pillsbury croissant dough. Baked until the crust is brown and the inside is all melty. Have you heard the term "kindred spirit"? Tanya is totally mine.

There was really no point beginning our reading knowing that the oven timer would be ringing in a few minutes. So we drank our wine and waited for the ding. We're a bit like Pavlov's dogs that way. We hear the oven bell and we drool automatically.

When our snack was ready, we put it in the middle of a large plate and poured crackers all around the outside. They were light crackers, baked, not fried, of course. The idea is you dip the crackers in the melted cheese. With your closest friends, you can really dig into the dip without feeling embarrassed. If your cracker doesn't at least threaten to break, then you don't have enough dip on it yet. That's my theory.

Eating all that cream cheese made us thirsty so we refilled our wine glasses. It was early, so we filled them to the top this time. There's just something about wine and cheese. I started to read the first sheet aloud. Adriamycin. Kind of a nice name. Adria for short. In fact, wasn't that a Sarah McLachlan song? ("Adria, I'm empty since you left me…" Close enough.) Bright red in colour. That's okay. I love the colour red. So far it didn't sound *that* awful.

Mistake number one: We read on. Side effects. I knew that hair loss would be a definite side effect of my chemotherapy treatments. I had been told that my hair would likely fall out quite quickly, sometime soon after the first cycle of treatments. Losing hair is always the big side effect that you hear about. I guess that's because it's the one that everyone can *see*. When you see a bald person, especially a woman, you think cancer. I do, anyway. I had not considered that hair loss *in addition to* a host of other side effects might be a reality. The side effects ranged from mild to severe and gave me chills. My mouth was dry. Time for another drink.

I can't remember at what point exactly Tanya brought the large wine bottle out and set it on the coffee table, but she did. It's one of those things that "just happened". It was the right thing to do. Definitely. The more wine we drank, the funnier mouth sores sounded. And heart palpitations. And rashes. And bleeding gums. And vomiting. And nausea. And so much more. My poor, sober husband looked on from the other couch. He clearly didn't see the humour in it.

We never really did finish reading that information. Maybe it would be better to go in to our meeting with open (empty) minds. Not all cluttered by too much specific information. Plus, we needed rest. Yes, that was what we'd do. We'd get a good night's sleep and jot down some questions in the morning.

Large half-and-half in one hand, pen in the other, Tanya began note taking as I thought aloud. Question number one: Why me? Number two: What the f%!&*? Number three: Is it okay to drink alcohol while on chemotherapy? We may have written down a few other questions, but not many. It's actually extremely difficult to formulate reasonable questions about something as utterly unbelievable and terrifying as chemotherapy.

So we were ready and waiting at the door when Shelley pulled up. We hopped in her car and set off on another cancer-related adventure.

Chapter 26:
Our Teaching Day with Nurse Judy

Secrets of the Bra-Bra Sisterhood

The drive was uneventful and we arrived early for our teaching session. We were taken to a small, comfortable meeting room. We sat and waited. Tanya said that the cancer centre wasn't really a place she imagined us going to together. Maybe Canada's Wonderland or Niagara Falls, but Juravinski? She decided then and there that she'd be in charge of planning the itinerary for our next visit. Good call.

In walked Judy. That smile of hers. It's very warm and welcoming. She's the kind of woman who automatically puts you at ease. If you ever have to talk about chemotherapy, call Judy. Just tell her Marcie sent you.

We did introductions and got down to business. Judy proceeded to answer every question I asked. (Yes, a glass of wine now and then while on chemo would be fine.) I saw Tanya quietly taking notes as she listened (Alcohol: _YES_). Earlier that day we had voted on who would do the writing, and it was unanimous. Tanya was elected. Her printing was the neatest and she was a nurse. She was the obvious choice.

Judy spent some time going back over my cancer history, explaining once again in simple terms about my specific type of cancer; the stage (two), the grade (three), the hormone receptor status (negative), and the Her2nu status (negative). Next, she moved on to the big topic of the day: chemotherapy. Specifically, A.C.T.

We learned that this type of chemotherapy, the kind that is given after a surgery such as a lumpectomy, is called adjuvant therapy. I was receiving chemotherapy for two reasons. First, it was important to get rid of any tiny, microscopic cancer cells that may have found their way out of my breast. We did not want any metastatic cancer (breast cancer cells that spread beyond the breast), that's for sure. Also, I was very young. It was necessary to be as aggressive as possible in our attempt to keep cancer away for as many years as we could. The younger you are when diagnosed with this disease, the more years you have to try to remain cancer free.

Next, Judy produced a very detailed calendar, marked with each of my chemotherapy dates, and reminders to take my various chemo-related medications on specific days. I would be receiving strong anti-nausea medications a couple of days before and after each chemo treatment. One was a strong steroid. I was hopeful that not only would the steroids keep my nausea and vomiting at bay, but that I might also become the athlete I had always dreamt of being. Lance Armstrong was going to get a run for his money! Sadly, it turned out the steroids I would be receiving were not the muscle-building type. Rats. You'd think there'd be at least some fringe benefits.

We received invaluable information that day from Judy. It was like talking to a friend. It was as if she could really relate to what I was going through. I felt as though Judy understood my fears. It was almost like she *knew*. Then she told us. Judy was a two-time breast cancer survivor. It just goes to show, you can't tell from looking at people whether or not they are survivors. Talk about a person giving me hope and strength. Her disclosure of this personal information completely explained Judy's ability to empathize with my situation (that and the fact that she's just a really fantastic person in general).

While breast cancer does not discriminate, affecting women young and old, people of all ethnic backgrounds, sexual orientations, even some men, there is one thing all breast cancer survivors have in common: We *know*. We all *know* the terror. We *know* the sleepless nights. We *know* the bargaining with some higher power. We *know* what it is to look death in the eyes and say, "No! If you want me, you'll have to come and catch me."

I am thankful to Judy to this day for being so open and honest, for sharing her personal story with me and for making my own experience much less frightening and isolating. I was certainly not alone. A bittersweet reality.

This feeling of solidarity, of a kinship with other women who have experienced, are experiencing or will experience breast cancer at some point in their lives, is something that grew during my journey to beat breast cancer. There is a combined strength in the knowledge that you are part of something larger, a sort of sisterhood of strong and courageous women. They are women with whom you can share good times and bad. I would be lucky enough to meet many of these women along the way and am grateful for their support, strength and humour during a difficult time. I feel that I can now pass on some of that strength to others during their journey. Together, we will overcome.

Chapter 27:
My First Chemotherapy Treatment

Chemopalooza #1

If I had been able to eat anything on the morning of my first chemotherapy treatment, I'd have been heaving it up in a big way by the time we got into the car to drive to Hamilton. Sometimes the body just knows when not to eat. This was one of those times. Then again, I wondered if having chemotherapy on an empty stomach was such a good idea. If taking over-the-counter medications on an empty stomach caused problems, what would full-on toxic chemicals do to me? Time would tell.

My husband and my sister were with me, but we drove in silence. It's not as if we could really talk about everyday things. Also, if any of us opened our mouths to talk, we knew there was every chance the bile would get out. So, the trip was long and quiet.

We pulled into the large, pay parking lot beside the Juravinski Cancer Centre. We got out. We walked to the front doors of the centre. We entered. We turned an immediate right and walked into the blood lab, as we had been instructed to do. I ran my health card through the computer and took a number. There weren't many people ahead of me. I had really been hoping to be number one million sixteen thousand or something like that. I think I was about 32, and they were calling 31 when I got there. Great time for my luck to change.

A nurse called my number and I followed her into the next room. It was very bright and clean. Not terrifying, really. There were several large, comfortable chairs lined up with little tables beside each. I sat down, trying to act really cool, as if this was just something I did sometimes for fun. Yep, just here to give some blood, then I think I'll head to Lime Ridge Mall and buy myself some new jeans. Act natural.

The nurse asked me if I had a preference for which arm to give blood from. Neither, I thought, but I went with the right. I'm not even sure why. I think it's partly because I had already decided that my left arm would be a better "chemo" arm. My right arm was still recovering from the lymph node dissection and felt tingly, numb and sometimes sore. So, it could be my "blood lab arm", leaving my left arm to handle the heavy stuff, like chemotherapy.

Thankfully, I have never had a fear of needles. As far as icky medical procedures go, needles have always been do-able. I realized early on in my life that if I didn't actually watch the needle going in, it was a piece of cake.

I rolled up my right sleeve (being new at this, I hadn't thought to wear a t-shirt for easier access to my veins) and proceeded to look around the room. Nice lighting. Friendly nurses. Interesting layout. Very good choice of chairs. Shiny floors. Ouch. Done. See? It's that easy.

One adventure down. One biggie to go. Next stop, Clinic D. We had been told to sign in after the blood lab at Dr. Tozer's clinic. Again, I handed in my health card. Perhaps today was the day that I should insist on being called Marcie Nolan. I *was* married, after all. I toyed with the idea of ignoring anyone who called out the name "Marcie Adams". That way, I wouldn't have to face whatever was coming next. That poor Marcie Adams. Wouldn't want to be her right now.

Shelley, Jeff and I sat in the familiar waiting room of Clinic D. We had waited there on the day we met Dr. Tozer and nurse

Judy for the first time. I have to say, it's much brighter and more comfortable there than anything I could have imagined for a cancer centre. Whoever designed and decorated that place had the right idea.

We managed to talk and probably even laugh while waiting. My name was called and once again I was led to the elephant scale. At least this time Dana was on the outside, so my weight had to have come down. We must find the positives where we can.

Still, I kicked off my shoes, set down my purse and spat out my gum. Then, slowly, I stepped on the mammoth-sized scale. Have you ever thought that getting on a scale really slowly, almost like sneaking up on it, would work in your favour weight-wise? Well, it doesn't, just so you know.

From the scale, I was led down the hallway to a small but comfortable waiting room. I awaited Dr. Tozer, breathing deeply and pretending to flip through an old Chatelaine magazine. Hmm, I think I'll try that homemade vegetable soup recipe as soon as the retching and dry heaving lets up.

Knock knock. A familiar face: Dr. Tozer. He came right in and smiled, putting me at ease instantly. Some people just know how to instill trust immediately, and he did that for me. It was almost as if he had met other cancer patients before me.

He explained that he had received my blood lab results and all was well. They had needed to check my white blood counts to make sure I was strong enough to receive a chemotherapy treatment. Chemotherapy kills white blood cells all through the body, so if you start off with a high count then your body can afford to lose some. Since this was my very first chemotherapy treatment, there had been no reason to worry about my white blood counts. This blood test simply provided Dr. Tozer with a number to compare the others to in the future. I was good to go.

Lucky me. My oncologist explained to me what would happen next and where I needed to go. Second floor. Chemo suite. How bad could a *suite* really be?

For some reason, it took us about five hours to get from Clinic D to the chemo suite on the second floor. Or maybe it just seemed that way. Regardless, we eventually found the reception desk and handed the receptionist my folder, the one that Dr. Tozer had sent with me. She took a paper from it and told me to pop the folder into the slot on the door up the hall. I did. Then, she handed me a number and told us all to sit down and wait for my number to be called.

The large open waiting area was welcoming. Not too creepy. We sat together all in a row. We spent some quiet time looking around. I know we were all noticing the numerous patients, all there waiting for chemotherapy. We saw men and women. Young and old. All shapes and sizes. Somehow in my mind's eye, everyone in the waiting room was much older than I. Yet, in reality, I was struck by the fact that cancer affects *everyone*. It is not only an old person's disease.

We saw people with all their hair. People with sparse hair in patches. People with absolutely no hair. People with wigs. People wearing head wraps. People wearing headscarves. People looking around. People with their eyes closed. People there with family and friends. People all alone. People. Regular people just like me. People who had been going along, living their lives and making their plans for the future when *poof*, their old life disappeared, making way for what we had come to call "the new normal". It just didn't seem fair.

I was reassured by the fact that I had been given number 23. I had often been warned by people to prepare for very long waits in the chemo suite. Sometimes hours. We had come prepared with food that none of us could even look at much less eat, trashy magazines by the dozen, novels (yes, I'm sure chemo would be a great place to really concentrate on a good plotline) and drinks (vodka would have been helpful at that time, but no one had had the foresight to pack any; water would have to do).

A nurse in a white lab coat walked into the waiting area and called out number 67. Interesting, given that I was number 23. I wondered if there were different number systems depending on what kind of cancer people had or what specific kind of chemo they were receiving. Shortly after that, number 8 was called. Then number 91. What the hell? It slowly dawned on us that the numbers were in totally random order and we had no idea how long we would have to wait. How cruel and unusual is *that*? For the love of God, I need order!

We relaxed and surrendered ourselves to the fact that we would likely be there a while. You can't stay on high-alert forever. Shelley noticed a volunteer at a little desk. She had "visitor" passes. Shell walked over and spoke to the lady. She signed a sheet, was handed two visitor's passes, each with a string to go around the neck, and returned to her seat with us. She handed Jeff a pass. They each put them on. Who knew it would be so easy to get a backstage pass?

Shell had been told that only one visitor was allowed to go into the chemo suite at a time with each patient. The two of them could trade off, one going in and the other staying in the waiting room. I had visions of my husband and my sister, each fiercely protective of me and desperate to be there with me for my first terrifying injection of chemotherapy, rolling around on the floor, fighting it out to see who would go in with me first. I admit that part of me wanted to see who would win. Then I wondered if, realistically, Jeff would simply let Shelley win so he wouldn't have to go in there.

As it turned out, neither one had the energy (probably from lack of sleep and food) to argue, so the decision was quickly and, I must admit, disappointingly easily made that Jeff would go first and Shell would join me halfway through. We had been told that each of my first four treatments, the Adriamycin and Cyclophosphamide parts, would take about one hour to inject. So, it was settled. Now all we needed was for my number to be called. I just wanted to get in and get it over with. Number 84? Oh good. I bet I'm next.

When at last my number was called, we all jumped. Shell hugged me and wished me luck. I can't imagine what was going through her mind as she watched me walk away, turning the corner and out of sight. I have often thought that it must take as much strength to be with someone as they go through a cancer diagnosis and all that it entails as it takes to go through it yourself. I don't know. It sucks either way. Still, I admire my sister for how well she handled each step of this ordeal. The thought of watching her go through this nightmare is worse for me than going through it myself.

Chapter 28:
Chemo on Our
Fifth Wedding Anniversary

Toto, we're not in Cuba anymore

Jeff and I followed the chemo nurse. She led us around the corner and I know we were both anxious to see what lay on the other side. Surprisingly, we entered a large, very bright open room. There were many windows and it was a sunny day. There were several big Lazy Boy chairs. The nurse asked me which chair I'd like to sit in. A chair in a pub somewhere would be nice, but probably not an option. So, I studied the room carefully.

Most chairs were empty. There was an elderly man in one chair, dozing with his eyes closed. Across the room my eyes landed on the only other patient in the room, a young, beautiful, vibrant-looking woman who was as bald as the day she was born. She wore a bright pink shirt and was already hooked up to her IV. Her chair was pushed back and her legs were outstretched on the footrest.

I noticed immediately that the corner chair, directly beside The Pink Lady's, was free. It sat in a beam of sunshine. I was drawn to The Pink Lady and I couldn't explain why. I wondered briefly if it would seem bizarre for me to pick a chair right beside her, when all around the room were empty chairs in much more private places. I went with my gut feeling and pointed to the corner sun-nook. If the chemo nurse was surprised by my choice, she did not show it.

I sat down and tried to relax. Impossible. I told the nurse I'd like the IV in my left arm, please. I rolled up my left sleeve. She sat beside me on my left side in a rolling chair, the kind I later learned was off limits to visitors for fear of injuries. Too bad; everyone would rather sit in a rolling chair.

The nurse was very kind and calm. Clearly, she had done this before. She explained what she would be doing and how it would work. She offered me juice, water and a cup of ice chips. Again, no mention of vodka. I said yes to all that she offered me, unsure of what I would want or need once we got going. She asked me if I had taken my anti-nausea medications two times per day, starting two days before my chemo day. Yes, I had taken them all, thanks to the constant reminders from my sister. Thank God for sisters. Well, for *my* sister, anyway.

Jeff sat on my right side, pale, bedraggled and powerfully supportive. This was a nightmare I'm sure he could not have dreamt up in his wildest imagination. I saw in his eyes deep love, fear, concern and signs that he was possibly about to choke on his own vomit. God love him.

This was not the way he and I had envisioned spending our fifth wedding anniversary. Yes, I am not making this up. It was July 22nd, our fifth anniversary. Most couples go on a trip, a date, out for a fancy dinner. We had fantasized about going back to our honeymoon resort in Varadero, Cuba. Not to chemotherapy. It was as though we were in an alternate universe. It occurred to me that a cancer diagnosis could either make or break a marriage. I was determined that this would make us stronger as a couple. Cancer would not ruin our "happily ever after". We held hands tightly and I knew that we were in this together.

Chapter 29:
More about Chemotherapy

You can't push me around!

My IV was hooked up without complication. I would be receiving Adriamycin first, right after a small pouch of anti-nausea medication. The Adriamycin was a bright red drug in a huge syringe. The nurse would do what was referred to as "pushing". At that point, it was kind of a relief that someone else had to do the pushing for a change. I'd had Dana. No more pushing for me.

She would attach the syringe to my IV and slowly, slowly "push" the drug through the syringe and into my vein. This was an extremely powerful drug and the body could only take so much at a time. My nurse had warned me to expect a metallic taste in my mouth instantly as well as a rush of freezing cold through my arm. She suggested I chew on ice chips and drink lots of water the entire time. Frozen ice chips would help with the awful taste commonly associated with this drug.

Sure enough, at the exact second that the Red Devil entered my vein, I could taste metal. Not vaguely. Not a slight hint of it. It's how I imagine chewing a big mouthful of tinfoil would taste, only worse. The taste made me gag and shiver, as I stuffed my mouth full of ice chips. Concentrate on chewing. Concentrate on chewing. Concentrate on chewing.

Also instantly, a cold rush up my arm. It's a shocking and scary thing, to feel a powerful drug entering your body. Talk about being helpless and out of control. I sat back and let the chemotherapy invade my body's cells. Better that than more cancer invading my cells. From the time I knew I would be receiving chemotherapy treatments, I had made a conscious choice to consider chemo my friend, a good thing necessary to help me in my battle against breast cancer. It was like strong armour in a war I was forced to fight. Why fight it unarmed? Chew. Chew. Chew.

Soon enough the red syringe was empty and I had successfully been treated with my first dose of Adriamycin. I had survived. The chemo nurse warned me to expect bright red urine a time or two when I was done. Good to know. I can imagine that after my first chemo the sight of bright red urine would have caused my heart to explode, hence causing even more problems I didn't need. Note to self: bright red urine is fine.

My next medicine, Cyclophosphamide, was a clear liquid in a pouch, hung on my IV pole. The nurse suggested I put my seat back and my feet up for the remainder of my treatment. She offered me a hot blanket. The worst was over.

Cyclophosphamide was not associated with the tastes and sensations of the Red Devil. The nurse simply hooked it up and left Jeff and me to ourselves. She assured me that she would not be far away if I needed her. We had about half an hour left, and we'd be walking out of there.

Chapter 30:
My First Chemotherapy Friend

Pretty in pink

While we sat and talked, we kept our eyes on The Pink Lady in the chair beside mine. She was chatting to her visitor, smiling and laughing. She looked so *healthy*. How could such a young, healthy-looking woman have *cancer*? What was she doing here? I managed to look at her for just long enough to make eye contact. She said hello and asked me what such a young, healthy-looking woman was doing getting chemo. I said that I had been about to ask her the same thing.

She introduced herself as Mary. When all introductions had been made, The Pink Lady told us that it was her third of four AC treatments. After her fourth treatment, she would be starting Taxol, just as I would be. Her breast cancer had been found in a routine mammogram. She had had her breast removed and was wearing a prosthesis. You'd never know it.

I told them my own story and we bonded instantly. It gave me such hope just looking at Mary. She was managing the chemotherapy treatments amazingly well, still living her life, proudly going bald at times and other times wearing bright, eccentric hats. Let me tell you, this woman made "bald" work.

I was comforted to know someone in the same boat as me, rowing merrily along, not sinking and drowning from the weight of the experience. While Mary was realistic and up-front with us about the difficulties and stresses of her journey (she and I both *hate* the word journey!), never making light of the realities she was enduring, she still managed to laugh and find humour in the little things along the way. I quickly decided she was "my people".

Chapter 31:
My Chemotherapy Cheerleaders

Halfway there

Jeff and I realized that we were about halfway through my first treatment. It was time for him to trade off with Shelley. If he didn't get out of there soon, she would come to us, and the fight I'd been rooting for earlier would take place. I have to say, Jeff basically ran out of there as soon as I mentioned that Shelley would be ready to come in. He'd been there to see me hooked up, held my shaking hand through the Red Devil's attack and had seen me connect instantly to a woman who would surely make my stay much more bearable. His work there was done for the time being. There was a toilet somewhere with his name on it.

As soon as Jeff was out of sight, my sister appeared. She walked over to my chair and had a seat. I told her about the Red Devil, the taste, the cold sensation and then introduced her to my new friend-for-life, Mary. As I knew they would, Mary and Shelley hit it off famously. We all love to laugh, to talk and generally choose to focus on the positives where cancer is concerned. I had already tried crying in the fetal position but had found that when I re-emerged, the cancer diagnosis remained. So, might as well have some fun along the way.

Shelley, being both my sister and my surrogate mom, offered me snacks, brought me more ice chips and found a new hot blanket to replace my now cooled-off one. Everyone needs to be pampered and taken care of in times of stress and fear, and my sister is the best nurturer and spoiler this world has ever known. In the arena of sisterhood, I'm certain that I got a better deal than she did.

Chapter 32:
Post Chemo #1

From the pink lady to the pink elephant

I had spent so much time thinking and worrying about my first chemotherapy treatment that I had never given much thought to what would come *after* it. When my IV machine beeped, indicating that my bag of Cyclophosphamide was empty, the nurse came over, unplugged it, popped on a new bag of clear fluid and told me it was just a quick "rinse". No more heavy chemicals for my system today. In 15 minutes my rinse was complete. My IV was removed. A band-aid was put on. I was free to go. Have a great day. See you in three weeks for Chemopalooza #2. How bizarre is that?

I got up, stretched and walked out of the room. On my way past the receptionist's desk, I was handed an appointment sheet that indicated when I was due back to the blood lab, Clinic D and the chemo suite. Exactly three weeks from that day. It should have been a bigger relief to be done, but the thought of doing this over and over again for six months was daunting. One day at a time. One day at a time. Let go and let God.

We got into the car and began the drive back to Guelph. Back to a reality we were more comfortable with. But first, we needed food. It's amazing how quickly an appetite can return after a stressful situation ends. I know that lots of people are unable to eat well during chemotherapy, but I was never one of them. My love of food knows no bounds. I like to think of my hearty appetite as a good thing, ensuring that I will never waste away. Nope, no fear of that anytime soon.

Jeff found a spot near the door and we happily, almost drunkenly, walked into Wendy's. A nice light lunch. Have you ever noticed that no matter how hungry you are you never crave a salad? I ordered a burger and fries, with a Coke. I was willing to deal with the consequences later, if necessary.

That moment felt like a celebration. I was now walking around with chemicals coursing through my body, cancer cells (if there were any hiding in there) being rapidly destroyed. Go get em', chemo! We ate and talked and laughed. We felt like ourselves again. Except we all knew we were about to go home and shave my head bald. Talk about a big pink elephant in the room. Who was going to mention it first?

Chapter 33:
Shaving My Head

Shave and a haircut...

We pulled into the driveway and parked. Home sweet home. Shelley and Jeff lugged the big chemo backpack full of uneaten snacks, untouched bottled water and unread magazines. I ran to the door, anxious to see my baby. My dad had been on Dana-duty while we were away. Imagine having to leave your three-week old baby for an entire day. It was hard, but something I had been psyching myself up for since before Dana was born.

We had sent Bryn to her babysitter, Dianna, earlier that morning. That was the best way to keep her routine constant. Besides, Bryn adored Dianna. Actually, we all did. Still do. She has been extremely helpful and flexible from my diagnosis on, offering to take Bryn even on her Fridays off and never putting pressure on us to decide which days we'd need her and which days we'd want to keep Bryn with us at home. She knew that throughout my months of chemo, we'd have no choice but to play it by ear, doing things according to how well I was feeling. We rested much more easily knowing that Bryn had a strong, loving bond with Dianna. Dianna's house had always been a fun, safe place to be. There were days when I'd drop Bryn off at Dianna's and wish that I could stay there, too.

After hugging Dana tightly and spending some time simply smelling her bald, round head, we put her down for her nap. Dad had picked Bryn up early to spend some time with her before we got home. She was ready for a nap, too. Good timing. We tucked the girls in and could put it off no longer. The pink elephant would not be ignored.

I had made the decision long before beginning chemotherapy that I would shave my head, or have Shelley do it, before my hair started coming out on its own. Partly, it was a control issue. I couldn't keep my hair from falling out, but I could control how it happened. Plus, the thought of my hair coming out a bit at a time, falling in my food, on my pillow, in my eyes, on the shower floor, made me feel physically ill. I had short hair to begin with, so maybe the change would not be *as* shocking. However, short hair by choice and bald by circumstances beyond my control are two different things.

Jeff and I had spent time talking to Bryn in what we hoped was an age-appropriate way about my upcoming chemotherapy and impending loss of hair. Things you never want to talk to your not-yet-three-year-old about. We had explained the "cancer booboo" at the time of the lumpectomy. As I continued to recover from that, Bryn was aware that mommy was still in some pain and had to be careful. We certainly didn't harp on it, but it was a reality in our household at that time.

The next step, we explained to our toddler, was for mommy to take special medicine called chemotherapy to help fix the cancer booboo. Mommy's special "chemo" medicine was so strong that it would make her hair fall out. When mommy's hair fell out, it meant that the medicine was working and doing its job well. How exciting! Gag.

Bryn was intrigued. It was, of course, a lot for a little girl to grasp. Much of the time we felt that *we* still didn't understand what was happening to me. How could we expect her to get it? She asked a few questions and accepted our simple answers. It appeared that she understood that my hair would all come out soon.

We tried to let her know, however, that I would still be me. The special medicine might make me extra sleepy sometimes, but mostly I would continue to take her out to play, do puzzles, share meals and spend time with our family. "You can wear pretty hats, mommy! So can I!" exclaimed my darling girl. Yes, we would wear hats together, I promised.

With both girls sleeping, it was time to get the clippers. Shelley had brought her home hair kit. It was a beautiful day and we figured outside on the deck was the perfect place for a de-hairing party. That way, we could just sweep the hair off the deck and never speak of it again.

Jeff stood by me, supporting and encouraging me to go for it. He shyly asked me if I'd like him to shave his head too, in an act of solidarity. His relief was palpable when I assured him that, while it was a sweet and brave idea, it was altogether unnecessary. Explaining to Bryn why mommy and daddy were *both* bald would be brutal. Besides, I wasn't totally convinced about the shape of his head under that hair.

My dad stayed to join the party. He and Shelley set me up a chair, got me a towel to keep the hair off my clothes and helped me get settled. Jeff brought out the digital and video cameras. He got a wine cooler for Shelley and me to share. Even I knew it wasn't a great idea to drink much alcohol on my very first day of chemotherapy. My liver had enough to deal with. So we split the cooler, neither of us finishing it, but both needing the comfort of it being there. It seemed to be the only thing we could cling to in order to call this thing a party.

What the neighbours were thinking is beyond me. Poor buggers, sitting on their decks having a BBQ while the sound of the electric clippers buzzed in the breeze. Yes, we were "those" neighbours. Jeff got a Guinness for himself, drank at least half in one terrified gulp and then took a couple of "before" pictures.

Shelley started the clippers and very quickly found that my hair was too long and thick for the clippers to work. It would be quicker, she decided, if she used a razor instead. So, I went in the house and returned with a head full of shaving cream, I'm sure to my neighbours' horror.

How can I describe the feeling of that first loss of hair? A loss. That's exactly what it was. For all my talk about being a confident person and woman, hair or no hair, losing my hair immediately symbolized a loss of part of me.

We laughed and joked as we watched chunks of hair fall away, but I can't say it was a completely festive occasion. I believe everyone shared my feeling of loss that day on the deck. There was an unspoken understanding that we were all wearing our brave faces because this had to be done, but no one would have wished it on their worst enemy.

In the end, we decided that shaving my hair down to the very shortest buzz-cut possible was enough at that time. I was just this side of bald, but it would be nice to take my time getting used to this look. Sinead O'Connor made it work. So did Demi Moore in the movie GI Jane. I would, too.

I'm sure Shelley wondered, at that time, how she had suddenly become the long-haired sister, her own super-short hair suddenly seeming to be a long, flowing mane next to mine. I bet she did not see *that* coming!

As a loving gesture, my dad sat down in the barber's seat after Shelley finished my shave. He had lost much of his hair years ago, but wanted what was left of it to be shaved off completely. What do people do without this type of support around them? We joked that it wasn't much of a change for dad to go from almost bald to bald, but in reality it was huge.

It was the act of a father who felt out of control and terrified; it was his way of going through this with me and of letting me know he'd do absolutely anything for me. With my turbulent teen and early-adult years long behind me, I am honestly able to say that I picked the right father. I don't dare ask him if he feels that way about me!

I spent a lot of time touching my fuzz. I was hyper-aware of my appearance and, although I have never been a high-maintenance person, I found myself constantly drawn to mirrors around the house to stop and look at the new me. It took a long time to get used to the look completely. There were many times when I would walk past a mirror and be startled by the stranger looking back at me. I admit that, at least in the early days, not only did I see a bald Marcie, I saw a *cancer patient*. It scared the hell out of me.

Talk about facing my fears *head*-on.

Chapter 34:
The Arrival of Our Favourite Nephew

It's a boy!

After the first chemotherapy treatment, there were three weeks until the next one. It was during the second week post-chemo, when I felt my best that the most incredible thing happened to our family. It got bigger. And so did our hearts.

For the past two years, my sister-in-law, Erin, and her husband, Brian, had been on a roller coaster of epic proportions. They had spent a two-week vacation in Haiti, volunteering at a foster home/school and helping out; Brian with repairs and Erin in the classroom. The fact that they chose to go on such a selfless trip was of no surprise to those of us who knew Erin and Brian well. They have never been people who sit around complaining about all that is wrong in the world. They are doers. Going to Haiti to make a difference was a natural thing for them to do together.

When they returned from Haiti at the end of two weeks, they had changed forever. Little did we know that Erin and Brian had truly made a difference while away. Not only did they teach children and improve the playground area at the school they visited. So much more had happened than any of us could ever have imagined.

It was not until a couple of months later that we found ourselves sitting on Erin and Brian's couch to hear all about the trip. Jeff and Erin's parents were there, too. A profound excitement was evident in Erin and Brian's eyes, in their body language and in their energy. Jeff and I both remember thinking to ourselves initially that it was a "work" vacation. How could they be so happy about that? We were thinking all along that they had been crazy (albeit extremely unselfish) to choose Haiti over, say, an all-inclusive resort in Hawaii.

The next thing that crossed our minds, as we listened to Erin and Brian share the details of their life-altering trip, was that maybe Erin was pregnant. You know how it is – anytime you know a happily married young, childless couple, you watch them like a hawk. Hmm, Erin hasn't had a glass of wine for a while. She does have a certain glow. I wonder…

Just when my curiosity was at a point where I wanted desperately to say something, to ask something that might trick them into sharing their secret, I saw a silent, meaningful glance pass between my sis-in-law and Brian. Fleeting, but real. Her eyes seemed to say that now was the time. His eyes agreed without hesitation. It *was* time.

I tried to hold in my excitement, ready for the baby news and hoping I'd be able to fake surprise when she told us. Erin cleared her throat and said, "Everyone, we have an announcement to make". Yippee! Jeff and I smiled at each other, that know-it-all, I told you so, kind of grin.

We have never been so right and so wrong at the same time in our lives! As the story unfolded, we learned that, while in Haiti, Erin and Brian had fallen in love. Big time. Not with each other (that happened years ago!). A gorgeous little boy named Max had stolen their hearts and had become a fixture in their lives and minds from the moment they laid eyes on him. No turning back. No turning away.

Jeff and I didn't know that Brian and Erin had privately discussed the idea of adopting a child long before this trip, but had figured they would wait a while, perhaps having a biological child or two first. So, it was not as shocking a decision as we may have initially believed. We had never discussed the topic of adoption with them and only knew that Erin and Brian would someday have children.

As surprised as we were at the news, we have always known that Erin and Brian were not a couple to rush into things without thinking, planning, and talking through the issues and concerns. Erin's a teacher, so you know she has thorough plans for everything! This particular plan, we understood, was not a knee-jerk reaction to meeting a lonely parentless little boy, but a natural next step after meeting the son they were put on earth to have, to raise and to love.

It was exciting to hear about our soon-to-be nephew, Max, through the emotionally charged words of his soon-to-be parents. We loved hearing Brian explain how, while planning the working vacation with Erin, he had spoken to her at length about the fact that they would be helping out at a school where many children did not have parents. This, he knew, would be extremely difficult for them both to see. He reminded Erin that, even though they knew they would someday adopt a child internationally, this trip was entirely separate from that plan. This vacation of sorts was their way of helping out, giving to others and bonding as a couple. Nothing could be better for a young couple. They had a bright future ahead of them, a future into which children would someday fit. Just not yet.

Brian was by no means cruel in his intentions to warn Erin about the children they were about to meet. He simply knew that she had a huge, kind heart and that upon seeing the little ones alone in the world, except for the wonderful staff at the school, her heart would break in two. You would have to be a monster to be able to see such a sight without at least entertaining the idea of rescuing them all!

Erin heard all that Brian had to say, patiently listening and nodding her head. Of course she understood and was as prepared as anyone could be for what challenges and joys awaited them in Haiti. She had by no means been secretly hoping to find "their child" while on this trip. Her goal was simply to be of service at the school, to get to know the children and adults, to encourage Brian to use his many skills to improve the schoolhouse and property surrounding it and, finally, to see first hand the Haitian way of life.

Part of the experience they had planned included them sleeping on site in a tiny room next to the rooms of the children themselves. This was not the kind of experience in which you could show up, help out a bit, and then return to a bright, spacious hotel room with a large tub and room service. Erin and Brian would live amongst the children and staff, helping with meals, eating beans and rice without seasoning, and sweltering in the heat. The smell of garbage surrounded them always, yet this was what they had signed up to do. They made the best of every minute of it.

Perhaps the best part of the story, as told by Brian and Erin about that first trip to Haiti, was what happened soon after their arrival at the school. They kept busy with their own projects, Erin using her experience as a primary teacher (and her knowledge of teaching French as a Second Language, since the kids at the school did their lessons and spoke mainly in French, not English). Brian, being the handyman and creative designer, fixed anything in need of repair, designed and built a new playground behind the schoolhouse and got to know the children as they followed him curiously.

Very soon upon arrival, Brian and Erin had met a handsome, sociable little boy with a grin from ear to ear. His name was Max and he loved people. He was quick with a joke and easily amused. Love, it seemed, and company, brought this little boy to life. Love and company, as it turned out, were things Brian and Erin had plenty of to share.

While helping Max and his classmates with the lessons each day, Erin had the opportunity to get to know him better. He was clearly a very bright child, learning quickly and with enthusiasm. He was hungry to learn, which made him the perfect student for his new teacher. I can picture the scene perfectly in my mind, as if I had been there to witness it all. Erin would be there, at Max's desk, speaking in French and also helping him learn English. The individual attention and opportunity to learn new information would make Max's eyes light up, sparkling as he looked into this woman's beautiful blue eyes. A love connection? I think so!

Almost immediately upon meeting Max, Brian was struck with a love he had not been prepared to feel. Perhaps it was the smile on that little boys face, or his laugh that could light up a room. It may have been his quick mind, his love of learning, or his openness with kind strangers.

This small child, only three years old, had lived through so much adversity in his short life, yet his heart remained open, his hope for a better life evident in all he did. Brian understood how easily Max could have shut down emotionally, how he could have closed his heart off to protect himself from further pain and disappointment. But that was not Max's way. He was strong and determined. I believe that Brian responded to that strength and determination in Max, sharing those traits and understanding that they were part of what connected them so quickly. Without realizing it at the time, Brian was going to need more strength and determination than at any other time in his life to bring his son home. But let's not get ahead of ourselves here.

Eventually, as you may have guessed, Brian approached Erin to talk in private. He spoke of the special paternal feelings he had toward Max, the little boy with the contagious smile. Erin, of course, didn't need her husband to convince her about their next step in life: They would adopt Max!

I wish I could have been a fly on the wall as they talked about Max openly for the first time, each one describing their feelings and hopes. Each one listing the pros and the cons of becoming his parents. Of course, it would not be an easy undertaking, to say the least. Erin and Brian knew little of the international adoption laws, particularly those in Haiti.

It had all happened so fast, but there was really no decision to make. They would adopt Max, bring him to Canada, raise him, adore him, parent him through all the good times and bad. Then and there, the commitment was made. All that remained was for them to return to Canada and contact a lawyer. If only they could have clicked their heels and magically brought Max home. Sadly, that was not the case.

After two long, heart-wrenching years of navigating through seemingly endless red tape, political turmoil, painful and joyful visits with Max, visits always ending too soon and with the hope that the next one would be to bring him home at last, the phone call came that made us literally jump for joy. Max was coming home! By this time, he was five years old, and he had never lived anywhere but in Haiti. As excited as he was to have parents and live in Canada, he would be saying goodbye to his friends, who were like siblings to him, and his schoolhouse. An exciting and terrifying adventure lay ahead.

Following the adoption laws of both Haiti and Canada, Erin and Brian headed to Haiti to spend several days with Max before they could pack up his few belongings, say their bittersweet goodbyes to the only family he had known thus far, and embark on a new life in Canada.

Needless to say, on the day of Max's arrival at the London airport where we would meet him for the very first time, we were overwhelmed with excitement, anxiety, joy, and all manner of other emotions depending on the moment. The balloons were up, the cameras were ready and we watched the airplane land. Hearts thumping, eyes straining to see the now-family-of-three exit the plane and enter our lives.

And then we saw *him*. Max. Gorgeous, perfect, smiling five year old Max with his proud parents, all holding hands as if they had been together forever. I admit that I could not hold up my camera to get many pictures of this once in a lifetime event. The tears streamed down my cheeks, blurring my vision entirely at times. I was literally shaking uncontrollably. My mind's eye still has all the pictures my camera didn't take, like a movie inside of me that I won't ever lose. I can replay every moment of that day in my mind at will. And I often do.

There was controlled chaos for a time, while hugs, tears, kisses, and more hugs were shared. Proud grandparents, aunts, cousins, Jeff the sole uncle, competed for Max and his parents' attention. It hardly seemed real after such a long wait. Could this little boy really be Max, my first and most precious nephew? I had seen pictures, talked to him on the phone, heard stories from Erin and Brian, but none of that was real. Not the way this flesh and blood person, tiny, overwhelmed, gorgeous and so very loved, was real. My eyes fill with tears even as I write of that magical day. The day our family grew and was instantly changed for the better.

I still can't imagine the range of emotions that Max must have experienced that day. The love he received. The overwhelming group that clamoured for him; the newness and strangeness of absolutely everyone and everything around him. If we were overwhelmed that day, our nephew could only have been blown away. As were his parents, no doubt. It will be interesting to see what Max's memories are of his arrival to Canada as he grows up. I feel so blessed to have the opportunity to be with him to find out.

A welcome home party at Erin and Brian's house followed our meeting at the airport. Oddly, it poured rain all the way to the airport that day, and continued pouring as we all ran to our cars to drive away, Max there with us. What a wet welcome he received to London, Ontario! Miraculously, or at least I like to think of it that way, it was a beautiful sunny day when we got to Erin and Brian's house. Max's house. Everyone was in the best mood possible. No way was a little downpour going to ruin our party.

Erin, Brian and Max were understandably exhausted, experiencing many emotions. The proud parents watched their son interact for the first time with his new family. Instantly, they were in the role of parents, only without the newborn, infant or toddler stages to prepare them for this active child of five years. Imagine getting to know your son for the first time as a walking, talking and very curious kid. Excitement aside, they were in for a long, hard road. Worth every minute of course, but difficult and exhausting all the same.

We, the extended family, were all on a high, beyond proud and relieved and thrilled to have our Max there before us in living colour. We, however, had not been in Haiti, on airplanes, and under the amount of stress that Erin and Brian had. It was much easier for us to let loose than it was for them. Really, as great as it was for us to welcome Max home ceremoniously, all that the new family of three needed was a long, long nap.

One of the many things that strikes me as amazing is that Max met me for the very first time as a bald woman. He had not known me before my cancer diagnosis. He had no memories of me as anyone but the woman who appeared before him at that first meeting at the airport. He accepted me instantly and happily, no judgments and no fear. I was simply Tante Marcie, his new aunt.

I do recall Max saying, upon meeting me, "Maman, Tante Marcie est tete-calle comme moi!" Yes, his mom replied with a smile on her face, his Aunt Marcie was bald like him. Max, you see, had been brought to the foster home as a baby with a head wound of unknown origin. It had been treated but left a permanent scar across much of the back of his head. The scar tissue that remains will never again grow hair. It was simply a child's observation that day, and thank God he was unaware of the reason for my baldness. At that time, I was the bald aunt who loved him. That was enough information for us both.

So, my nephew has a bald patch that is only one small part of him, the way some people have a mole, or freckles or wear glasses. We love him exactly that way. To be honest, I don't know if any of us ever even notices it anymore. It's hard to notice anything but his winning smile and huge personality. He is home. He is loved. He is respected. He is so much to so many. Did I mention that he is *home*? Home sweet home.

Chapter 35:
Preparing For the
CIBC Run for the Cure

Just do it!

I admit that I have never been much of a participator when it comes to charities. I've donated to good causes, written cheques to help out, but I've never gone beyond the most basic kind of giving; the financial kind. I can't say that it ever even crossed my mind to sign up for a run, a walk or a special event. I was busy. I had a life. It didn't really affect me personally. You see where I'm going with this.

Sadly, it often takes a personal tragedy or experience to make us look outside of ourselves and see the bigger picture. It's simple to have the "I'm just one person. What can I do?" mentality as an excuse to hide out and cop out. I know *I* did. Again, in my recent trend of learning by experience, I have come to realize that it is precisely those of us who are healthy and able who are so needed in the fundraising and charity events that raise money for more research. Just think of how many cures are out there, waiting to be found. If only there was more money.

My sister called me one day in early September to tell me about a special event she had heard about on the radio. It was called the CIBC Run for the Cure, a run to raise money for breast cancer research. She wanted to go online and register us as a team. She wanted to get the go-ahead from me to e-mail a bunch of our friends and family, outlining the details of the run and inviting them to join us as we marched toward a cure. Of course, suddenly I personally understood the importance of this event and encouraged her to go for it. I was in.

I was always the procrastinator in our family. Shelley, on the other hand, doesn't waste time. She gets things done. Fast. I believe that it was later the same day that I received an e-mail from the new CIBC Run team captain of *Mighty Mar and the Marvelous Marchers*. How cool a name is that? Shelley had sent it to many, many people and it was written in such a way that it made me proud, it made me excited, and it made me cry; all at once. Again, how did I get so lucky as to have *her* in my life?

The e-mail read:

Dear Friends and Family:

I hope that everyone has had an enjoyable and relaxing summer! It's hard to believe that fall is just around the corner. With that in mind, I would like to invite you to participate in the 14th annual Canadian Breast Cancer Foundation CIBC Run for the Cure on Sunday, October 2nd, 2005. The annual run/walk is held each fall with proceeds going to the Canadian Breast Cancer Foundation (www.cbcf.org) to fund breast cancer research, treatment and educational programs in Canada. With estimates that breast cancer will affect one woman in 9 during her lifetime, it is obvious how important this research is. Mar's diagnosis in late April has brought this issue very close to home as we have all seen first hand how she is dealing with her cancer with strength and determination (and lots of humour!). The goal is that women will no longer have to deal with this illness, and this walk gives us a way to contribute to the fight to end breast cancer.

To honour Mar and support her in her journey, I have registered a team for the run/walk called:

Mighty Mar and the Marvelous Marchers

I have enclosed an information package with details of the run/walk, and additional information is available at the above website. Please join Mar and me on October 2nd for some fresh air and fun, and together we can march toward an end to breast cancer!
Sincerely,
Shelley (aka Bug, aka Mar's sister)

PS. Please forward this to anyone else you think would be interested - the more the merrier!

Needless to say, in no time at all, our team came together. Every day Shelley heard from more and more people, women and men alike, who had gone online and proudly joined our team. It made me feel mighty just watching this strong support group encircle me with love. Mighty. Mighty *lucky*, indeed.

It is a strange thing, to watch a group of loved ones come together for *you*. To support *you*. To find *you* a cure. To try and save *your* life. It is extremely powerful. I recall knowing long before the actual run day that it was going to be an overwhelmingly emotional day. On many levels. Sometimes I would think about the day, picture it in my mind and the tears would well up. I would be surrounded by my favourite people, and we would we be walking for a cure to put an end to a hideous disease. I felt a chill when it dawned on me that I *needed* that cure. My God, I could die without it.

There is, or at least has been for me, a phenomenon that happens sometime during the breast cancer journey. Suddenly, you feel as though you have millions of "sisters". You become acutely aware of all the women who have died of this disease; who have gone before you. All the women who have fought *it* bravely, for better or worse. All the families that have sat by, helplessly watching their mother, wife, sister, grandmother, aunt, daughter, friend, partner die too soon. You are not alone.

There is a whole community of fighters, survivors, and, sadly, lost women; lost but never forgotten by the loved ones they have left behind. How can you not feel proud to be a part of something that is much, much bigger than yourself? Humbling and nourishing. Saddening and empowering. It is an honour to be a member of a club so full of brave women. A club that no one chooses to join, but once you are a member, you will be in it for life.

Chapter 36:
My Support Network

Near, far, wherever you are

Around the time that Shelley was organizing Team Mighty Mar and the Marvelous Marchers, I received an e-mail from Tanya in Halifax. She explained that she had gone online and registered her family as a team for the Halifax CIBC Run for the Cure. Did I mention the kindred spirit thing?

She asked me for permission to post a picture online of me, bald and beautiful, holding baby Dana (also bald and beautiful). She was accepting online donations and had composed a write-up about me that friends and family could read. A picture that would melt hearts and open wallets. I was all over that idea! And so my support group and the run team widened to include the Maritimes.

One of my dad's best friends, John Henry, who has been like an uncle to me over the years, showed up at my door one day for a visit. He had driven in from Mississauga just to see me. I opened the door to see John sporting a new, completely shaved, bald head. Man, the support was astounding. We definitely looked related now, hairless and proud of it!

Some people do things that really, really surprise me. I confess that, coming from John, the act of support and love, the shaving of his head for me, was far from surprising. Knowing

John as I do, with his big heart and big ideas, it would have been more surprising to me if he had *not* shaved his head. Still, I won't ever forget that he did that for me.

Daily, in that early fall as the big run approached, I received dozens and dozens of e-mails from people literally all over the world. They had heard about me from a friend, a relative, someone at their church, someone on their street, and they had begun praying for me. Daily. Me, a stranger to them. The prayers and love poured in by way of e-mail and it built me up to read the messages. There was even a group praying for me in Medjugorje, including a priest. He e-mailed me personally to show me a prayer card he had received. I accepted the prayers, thankful for love that I wasn't sure I had earned.

I had never reached out to a stranger that way, but would certainly do so from that point on. It really reminded me that people *can* be so good. In a world where we see and hear so much negativity, experiencing such pure, unselfish goodness was refreshing.

Speaking of unselfish goodness, upon receiving word of my diagnosis, my colleagues jumped in to help in a big way. Karen Whitworth and Pam Servos, teachers I had always enjoyed working and visiting with, showed up with boxes full of donated casseroles, stews, muffins, loaves, and so much more. The meals had been collected from all staff and administration at my school. Needless to say, we ate well at every stage of the game thanks to the staff at Brant Avenue Public School.

One of the most amazing, heart-warming (and fun!) surprises of all in the early days of my diagnosis was a "get well" shower thrown by my colleagues soon after my lumpectomy surgery. Instead of the usual baby shower theme, they had decided that the focus would be on me. Jill Mountford, another Brant teacher who is known for her wacky sense of humour, arrived with gift after gift, treat after treat, a huge garbage bag full of well-wishes from the gang at work.

Unfortunately, I was not home on the delivery day so Jill took the loot into my backyard. She was looking for a good place to hide the gifts, a spot to protect them from the rain that was coming down at the time. It did occur to her, she explained later in that hilarious Jill way, that the scene may have looked a bit shady to the neighbours. She was creeping around my backyard with a black garbage bag flung over her shoulder. Luckily, our policeman neighbour, Mike, was at work at the time!

She settled on the inside of our barbecue as the best place to leave the treasures. She did leave me a big note at the front door to let me know the gifts were back there. It would have been a crying shame if Jeff had gone out to warm up the barbecue one day, only to smell the burning offerings.

I sat and dumped the bag of gifts out on the floor. I spent the longest time just reading cards, opening thoughtful gifts and crying. I missed work. I missed my colleagues and their stories. I missed sitting on student desks after the kids had gone home for the day, swapping tales with Brent, Cara, Sylvia, Sarrah and so many others. I missed my old life.

Judging from the pile of magazines, bubble bath, scented candles, wine and many other goodies, I was missed at work, too. It felt good that I was gone but not forgotten in the work world. My friends at Brant continued to keep me in the loop as far as what was going on at the school. We e-mailed and I joined them once in a while for a Friday night drink and munchies. I was happy to have a connection to my work life while I was away.

The final surprise occurred when I received an e-mail from Sylvia Mollison, Grade 3 teacher and integral part of all things social. She wanted to know what weekend dates I had free in the next couple of months. She was going to throw me a baby shower! It would be at her house, and my kids (Dana had been born by that time) were welcome. Sylvia has two gorgeous children of her own, McKenzie and Parker. They would happily play with my girls if I decided to bring them along.

Given that my work friends had already been more than generous with gifts, food and support, the news of a baby shower for Dana came as both a shock and a thrill. My pregnancy with Dana had certainly been overshadowed by my cancer diagnosis and required treatments. Often I found myself mourning the loss of the full pregnancy experience.

Don't get me wrong; I'm no fan of actually *being* pregnant, but I really had wanted Dana; had planned for her to come into our lives, and felt guilty that her pre-arrival womb time had been spent without fuss. At a time when it should have been all about her, we were just happy we remembered to show up on her assigned due date!

The baby shower date was set and I looked forward to the fun. The Brant social committee knew how to throw a party! On the day of the big celebration, I arrived with both girls; one in my arms (crying and showing her colicky side, of course) and one by my side, clinging but also curious. Bryn got comfortable with Sylvia's kids soon enough and went off to play. Good, I thought. Now I could show off Dana, the reason for the party.

Which would have been great if Dana hadn't screamed like the spawn of Satan.

Every mother wants people to meet and fall instantly in love with her children. Or, I do, at least. Not so easy with a screamer. A crier. A yeller. A Gerber baby Dana was not. Cute? Yes. Smiling? Not so much. On baby shower day, my colleagues got to know Dana far more than they had ever wanted to, I'm sure. They kindly took turns passing her around, each one trying a trick or two they'd learned to calm her down. To no avail. I think it was around that time that I started drinking wine. It was also around that time that Dana either started to get a bit better or I started to care about it less. Coincidence? I think not.

I have to share with you that there was a pile of gifts literally up to the ceiling that day. As if the party had not been enough, there were gifts for both Dana and her proud big sister. We opened gift after gift, card after card. It was overwhelming. To look around the room, full of smiling colleagues, it was clear that everyone was happy for the chance to get together and celebrate something positive with me. I will never forget the gifts, the friendship and the immense support of my colleagues that day.

It pains me to admit that, as well meaning as I was, I never did get around to finishing all the thank you cards that sat, partially written, for days, then months, and sadly, now years. I suck. At this point, to simply say "thank you" seems terribly inadequate after the steady stream of support that I received, but I hope it's not too late to tell my colleagues what a difference they have made in my recovery and in my life.

Chapter 37:
Cathy's Big News

You look mighty fine in those mat pants

In the midst of plans for the big CIBC Run for the Cure, one of my best friends in the world received the greatest, most exciting news ever; Cathy was going to have a baby! When Cathy and her husband got married a year before, I had welcomed Mike as an honourary friend. You know that special relationship you hope to have with your friend's partner? I loved him for Cath and knew they were a strong team. Even then, I dreamed of their family-to-be. No pressure.

In a way, you'd think it would have been hard to have Cathy experiencing the best time of her life while I was at my worst, and yet the opposite was true. From the moment I heard Cath's news, I was elated. I had always known Cathy would be an amazing mother, and now, at last, her dream (and mine) had come true.

Many times when I felt down or defeated, I would simply close my eyes and try to imagine what Cathy's new little person would look like. Would it be a boy or a girl? I listed the best (or worst?) baby names to go with their last name, Pearce. How about Ear (pierce)? Or Nose (pierce)? The list went on and on. Remember, this big news came at a time when I was lying awake most nights for hours. Yes, lots of time on my hands, that's for sure. I was bound to come up with the perfect name for my, er, her, baby eventually.

There's nothing like the impending birth of a much-anticipated baby to give a person strength and courage (especially when the impending birth does not involve my feet in the stirrups). I now had one more major reason to fight this disease with all I had. I intended to be around to meet baby Pearce, to spoil this child, to watch this little person grow and change and become whoever he/she was destined to be. Someone great; of that I was certain. No, I wasn't going anywhere. My girls were going to have a new buddy to play with, and I had another excuse to go shopping in the baby section.

Chapter 38:
Back to Chemotherapy

Chemopalooza #2: Electric Boogaloo

After my first chemotherapy treatment, I never again felt as nervous and wretched as I had on day one. I had survived the head shaving and the various side effects, which so far had been relatively mild in nature. I had had mouth sores that disappeared as quickly as they had appeared and the taste of metal had lingered only for a few days. There was some stomach upset the day after chemo, but it was easily controlled by my anti-nausea pills. Other than that, I was still me.

I recall waking up in my bed the first morning after chemotherapy. I lay still. Very still. Yes, I was definitely breathing. A very good sign. Hand to shaved head. Creepy, but do-able. I sat up. Still fine. I walked around. Stretched. Nothing. How could I have just received chemotherapy not even 24 hours ago and feel exactly the same as I did before the chemo? Mind-boggling. It was a relief to still feel like myself. As long as my head wasn't in the toilet, I was happy. So far, so good.

On the morning of Chemopalooza #2, my appetite did not disappear. We hit the drive-thru at Tim's for coffee and bagels with cream cheese. I ate, drank and felt good. It looked as though we would be reading our trashy magazines that day, as we all had a much better sense of humour that time around.

Treatments two through four went by as easily as chemotherapy can go by. I don't pretend that it was no big deal. It was huge. I was increasingly tired and sore each time I went. I had a colicky newborn to care for, and at a time when nurses and doctors everywhere were telling me to get much more sleep than normal, I was getting up two, three and sometimes even four times each night to feed the baby.

Dana was not much of a daytime napper, either, so I was not catching up on lost sleep during the daylight hours. I was like the walking dead, only way more stubborn. Chemotherapy and cancer would not ruin my life. No time to crawl into a hole. Must keep mothering.

The beauty of the human mind is that it is astoundingly able to see the funny side of darn near any situation, or *my* mind can, at least. It is not really in me to feel sorry for myself for very long. I generally am able to find the humour in my life, even if I have to dig a little to get to it.

Take Chemopalooza number two, for example. I had requested a seat next to the Pink Lady, like last time. Mary and I are both creatures of habit, so were in the exact same seats as three weeks previous. We talked and laughed and had a grand time. If you could have heard us but not seen us, you'd have assumed we were two old friends at a restaurant having lunch. A good time was being had by all. Soon after we got to talking, Mary had a visitor. In walked a woman with a great smile and mischievous eyes. I liked her already.

Lee is Mary's friend and colleague. They work together, writing and editing for a local newspaper. Lee is also a breast cancer survivor, having completed her chemotherapy a few months before Mary began hers. Another hilarious Pink Lady? This chemotherapy thing was a laugh-riot!

It didn't take long for us to stumble onto the topic of chemo side effects, a topic we could all relate to on different levels. I was the newest chemo girl, so had a lot to learn from my more experienced pink friends. We laughed at the whole hair loss thing, especially the fact that you didn't just lose the hair on your head. Very funny, at least if you're in "Survivor" company.

My new friends found it hilarious that, while all of my hair had fallen out everywhere else, wouldn't you know I still had enough on my legs to have to shave them? Yes, there I'd be, sitting on the edge of my bathtub day after bloody day, as bald as the day I was born, but shaving my legs. Is there no justice in the world at all?

We also swapped stories about mouth sores, headaches and muscle pain as though we were talking about the weather. How quickly things can become routine. I found so much comfort in hearing Mary and Lee's stories. It was a rare thing for me at that time in my life to be among others just like me. Others who had also learned to laugh at the unthinkable. Other women who had been through it all, every step of the way, and had managed to come out laughing, at least most of the time.

The advice from the gals proved very helpful time after time. For example, Mary had already told me, at Chemopalooza number one, that she found ginger and buns very helpful to keep her mild stomach upset and nausea at bay. I had made a mental note: Ginger. Buns. Good to know.

After our first meeting, Mary had told Lee about her visit with Shelley and me in the chemo suite, although she couldn't remember our names. She explained that she had told me to take ginger and eat buns if my stomach got iffy.

Fast-forward to Chemopalooza number two. Lee was meeting Shelley and me in person for the first time, and remembering what she had heard about us from Mary. She asked me, "Which one are you? Ginger or Buns?" It turned out that Mary had been talking about us, calling us Ginger and Buns, until she could ask us our real names again!

I told Lee that I was Ginger, and Shelley was Buns. I couldn't tell you why I chose Ginger. It was just such a fun experience to have at a chemotherapy treatment. From that moment on, I have been Ginger (Gingerella, Gingerbread Cookie, Gin and Tonic, and all manner of other ridiculous nicknames) when in the company of my Pink Ladies. Chemotherapy is a lot of things, but if you open yourself up and are lucky enough, it is never boring.

Chapter 39:
My Maritime Mother Visits

The other glove

I couldn't have been happier, or more relieved, when Tanya, her 11-month-old son, Jacob, and her mom, Susan, arrived to help Jeff and me out with the girls, the house and all the little details of life that were becoming too much for us to handle on our own.

While living in Halifax as a child, I spent so much time with Tanya that we were like sisters. As such, we each had grown extremely comfortable in each other's homes and with each other's parents and siblings. We came and went freely from one house to the other, as if we each were members of both families simultaneously.

Looking back, I still remember feeling how much Tanya's mom loved me. I wasn't just some kid who lived up the street; a child who seemed to show up every other night at about dinnertime. I was like her daughter, in a way. We were close and I loved her.

After my mother died in 1993, Susan and I became even closer than we had been before. She never once tried to replace my mom in any way, but she gently let me know that she would be there for me in any way I needed or wanted her to be. We regularly exchanged phone calls and e-mails, letters and cards. Anytime I called to talk to Tanya, I would spend some time talking to Susan as well.

After losing my mom, I remember sharing a poem with Susan in an e-mail. It was one written by a Canadian poet named

Dorothy Livesay, one that I had read in a high school English class, jotted down and tucked away for safekeeping.

It had recently come back to me in the middle of the night while I lay awake, missing my mother terribly. I couldn't stop thinking about it and why, at that particular time of grieving, it had resurfaced in my memory.

The poem is called "Time" and it goes like this:

The thought of you is like a glove
That I had hidden in a drawer.
And when I take it out again
It fits; as close as years before.

I explained to Susan in writing what I was unable to say out loud. I admitted that every time I read or thought of my mom, I remembered that poem. I would spend hours at night recalling my mom's voice, her smell, her touch, her laugh; it always felt, briefly, as though she had never left me. The poem went around and around in my mind, along with visions of Nancy Elaine Adams. My mom.

There are events in my life that have forever changed me. Susan's response to my e-mail that night is one such event. She understood immediately the connection I felt to that poem. She knew how hard the loss of my mom had been for me and how I now clung to memories to keep my mother close.

I felt certain then, as I sat crying and reading her words, that Susan LeRue was in my life for a reason. She was special. And then I read how she ended her note to me. Tears filled my eyes as I read over and over again

Love always,
Susan (The Other Glove)

From that day on, Susan has really been the other glove in my life, that other mom I so desperately needed but felt too guilty to ask for. She found the perfect way to connect with me as my mother figure, without threatening my loyalty to my real mom.

Some people are not lucky enough to have one loving, caring, supportive mother in their lifetime. It amazes me still that I have been blessed with so many.

Chapter 40:
The CIBC Run for the Cure

Running for my life

On the morning of the CIBC Run for the Cure, many of us had arranged to meet at our friends' house. Monica and Dave Durbin live right downtown, so are usually the starting point for activities in that neighbourhood. I'm not sure if they thought about that when they decided to buy downtown. It can be a bit like Grand Central Station around their place sometimes. They graciously take us all in; offer us coffee and go with the flow. Don't you love people like that?

We assembled on their front lawn, babies in strollers, toddlers hand-in-hand (we have already decided that our Bryn and their Benjamin will get married as soon as they turn 18, so we encourage them to hand-hold regularly). Moms and dads with Tim's for the walk. Cathy had arrived the night before, pregnant, tired and every bit the cheerleader she has always been for me. So, there she was, running shoes on, baby bump visible, smile on face. And we were off.

It was a cool, crisp morning and it looked as though the sun was going to shine all day. We had ordered sun and God had delivered. The arrangement had been for those of us walking from the Durbin house to meet the rest of the Marvelous Marchers at the run meeting area. Clearly, we were all doing this for the first time. Mental note: when meeting several people for a charity event, pick a very, very specific place to gather.

Turns out, we were not the only team walking that day. The place was packed and I instantly felt the energy of the group. I'm not sure what I had expected, but this was far larger, far more powerful than my mind could have conjured up.

Eventually, we did piece together the entire team, one Marcher at a time, and Shelley, our fearless leader, went to pick up our team shirts and goodies. As I scanned the crowd around me, my breath was taken away. A sea of people, mostly women, all in white CIBC Run for the Cure T-shirts. Then I saw *her*. A bald, beautiful less-than-middle-aged woman in a pink t-shirt. Chills. All cancer survivors were given pink T-shirts for this event, to distinguish them from their supporters.

She noticed me as I noticed her and we connected instantly. She made her way through the crowd and gave me a big hug. We exchanged names and stories. She introduced me to her young children and I introduced her to mine. We were in this together. Another sister on my journey.

My teammates donned their white T-shirts and pinned on their bib numbers as well as their "I'm Running For_____" signs. They all ran for me as well as others they knew who had battled or were battling breast cancer. It was touching and heart-breaking to see Bryn, my little girl, with a tag that said "I Run For Mommy".

After official welcomes and motivational speeches, we were on our way. The crowd, thick at first, spread out as some people ran, some walked quickly, and others (us) rambled slowly but surely. We were not in it for a first place medal. We were just happy to be a part of something so amazing.

We talked, laughed and, at times, got choked up. Along the way, strangers in cars who were stopped at traffic lights, honked their horns and yelled their support out of windows. They waved, cheered and whistled for us. For *me*. I proudly wore my pink t-shirt and felt the breeze on my bald head. My head was held high that day and I was able to make eye contact without hesitation with everyone I met. This group was safe. This group *knew*.

By the end of the "Run" (I use the term "run" loosely, as the only running going on with our team was the constant running of toddler noses along the way), we were at the very end of the pack. One other woman, a fellow mom with her toddler, shared our spot as last but not least to finish.

When the finish line was in full view, my heart skipped a beat. There was a crowd, watching us, hollering for us. Eyes were on us. Teary eyes. I picked up my pace and ran the final steps to cross the finish line, arms in the air, victory in my soul. I was a champion at that moment and it felt amazing.

Some events are life changing. The CIBC Run for the Cure was one such event for me. For many, I believe. It gave me strength. It gave me hope. It gave me courage. It gave me love. What more can you ask for, really? I thank my friends and family for sharing that day, that soul-altering experience, with me. I thank my sister for signing us up and assembling the best team around. I thank CIBC and the Canadian Breast Cancer Foundation for making it all happen. I thank the folks at the Running Room for their sponsorship. I thank God that I have been blessed, yet again, in so very many ways.

Chapter 41:
Claudia Rebecca Durbin's Baptism

All in the family

In the midst of a difficult time, it's always nice to find an occasion to celebrate. In our case, the baptism of our goddaughter, Claudia Rebecca Durbin, was indeed cause to gather around with friends and family, and welcome her into the church community.

As Claudia's big day approached, Jeff and I became increasingly excited. We had a positive, emotional, heart-warming ceremony coming up and we wanted to look *good*. Jeff had his best suit dry-cleaned and ready to wear (he was, after all, the godfather, as he constantly reminded me in his best Marlon Brando voice). I, on the other hand, needed to go hat shopping. Big time. I wanted so desperately for the baptismal day to be all about Claudia. Me, standing before the congregation bald and puffy, was not an option.

I called my shopping partner, Shelley, and we headed to the shops of downtown Guelph. Guelph really is a beautiful city and its downtown is thriving. Lovely, unique shops and lots of interesting people going by. It was a sunny day and we were on a mission. Shopping is always great when you don't need anything in particular. You know how fun it is to be walking by a shop window and see "the perfect thing", the thing you didn't know you needed until the moment you saw it?

Well, it's a whole different scenario when you have two hours to find the perfect hat. Not that we were being picky. Our only criteria for the perfect "proud-godmother-going-to-her-gorgeous-goddaughter's baptism" hat was that it be black, understated, not too casual, not too dressy, no feathers, no lace, couldn't make my face look pale or puffy or fat, and must not make me look like a cancer-patient. If it happened to make my whole body look 10 pounds lighter, then all the better. Good luck with that.

Would you believe that we found exactly the hat I had pictured in my mind's eye? In a unique, homey store downtown that sells gently used clothing. Let it be our little secret that my dream hat cost a startling dollar to purchase. Yup, nothing's too good for my goddaughter! So I forked over my loonie and was on my way. I was going to dress up and go out into the world as a godmother, not a chemo-girl. No one would even be able to tell. This was going to be great!

At home, I washed my gently used hat twice. You never know what kind of head that hat lived on before mine. To be honest, it kind of made me itchy just thinking about it. It was, however, the perfect hat so I washed it obsessively and then put it on. Still perfect. Man, I looked good.

I awoke giddy on Claudia's baptismal day. My smile, I'm sure, went from ear to ear. It was an honour to be chosen to play this special role in Claudia's life. Actually, it meant more to us than we have ever been able to express. I went to my closet, pulled out my black slacks and burgundy top, grabbed the one black dress shoe that was on the floor and spent 20 minutes hunting down its mate. The hat was on my dresser, waiting to be used as the piece that pulled my whole outfit together.

And then I put my black slacks on. Well, I tried to. Several times. Unkind words were spoken. It seemed that my dress pants had shrunk terribly in the wash since I last wore them. Perhaps I should have tried them on before now. Note to self: never assume your outfit will be fine if you haven't worn it in several months.

I ran around in my panty hose (not really a good look, I admit. There must be a better expression than "spare tires"). Funny, the panty hose had shrunk, too. They must have been in the same load as the pants.

Eventually, I found a pair of nice black pants that had "stretch" on the tag. Thank God for "stretch", whatever that is. I was ready to go. Jeff looked very handsome and not at all like the mob king he was impersonating. I put on my pride and joy: the new hat.

Have you ever found the perfect clothing item and fallen in love? Then you get it home and find that it's nothing like what you thought it was? Some freakish mix-up must have taken place. That was precisely my experience with "the hat". It sat funny no matter what way I put it on. Its rim was very soft so was forever getting in my eyes. I was constantly aware of that damn hat. And I didn't look slimmer in it, that's for sure. Too late now. The show must go on.

We arrived at Dublin Street United Church in downtown Guelph. We met up with Claudia's parents, our good friends Monica and Dave. The ones whose home we forever gather at whenever anything is happening downtown. We were all ready for the big ceremony and Claudia looked absolutely perfect; a real Gerber baby if ever I've seen one. Can a godmother take any credit when her goddaughter is beautiful?

Benjamin, Claudia's handsome big brother (Bryn's husband-to-be), was also dressed up for the occasion. As he watched the group gather, he smiled his shy, Benjamin smile and I felt in my heart that all was well in the world.

The baptism was an amazing celebration. Claudia was welcomed into the church with loving, open arms. The members of the congregation promised to help guide her in her walk with Jesus. We, as godparents, vowed to help teach her our Christian values. We will do our best to always lead by example. Claudia deserves nothing less from us.

The party back at the Durbin house allowed friends, family, and loved ones with varied connections to Claudia and her parents, to mingle; to get to know one another better, and, of course, to coo over the baby girl we were all there to celebrate. Amazingly, amidst the hustle and bustle, the hat ceased to matter. When counting my blessings, the Durbin family ranks very high.

Chapter 42:
The Truth about Chemotherapy

Supersize me

As it turned out, my black slacks and panty hose were not the only items of clothing that had shrunk since I began chemotherapy. Anything I tried to put on from the waist down was disturbingly snug. Even my "fat girl pants", the ones I wore when very early in my pregnancy with Dana (too big for my regular pants, but not ready for maternity pants yet) seemed to have shrunk a good size and a half. No one wants to admit that she's outgrown her big pants.

When you picture a person on chemotherapy treatments, what do you see? For me, the image has always been that of a pale, emaciated person. Not a chubby, round around the edges, rosy-cheeked woman as I had clearly become. "Jolly" was the term Tanya used. In her defence, she used the term about us *both*. Very helpful Tanya. Thanks!

How had this happened? I have never had a weight problem (although I admit to many years of hating my body, obsessing about my weight and general discomfort in my skin) and I had been pretty much the same, healthy weight for years. How is it that literally one day I looked in the mirror and didn't recognize myself at all? No hair. Dark circles under my eyes. Puffy, perfectly round face. And a jolly body. Very helpful to my self-image as I came to terms with my lack of hair and cancer diagnosis in general. As if it wasn't hard enough without the fat thing.

OK, I confess to having some idea about how I got so jolly. There is a slight chance that the steroids in my chemotherapy drugs, combined with my absolutely sedentary lifestyle, the stress bingeing and the attitude that I had cancer and a newborn so I could bloody-well eat poutine three times a day if I so chose (and, sadly, I so chose pretty regularly over the course of my six months of treatments), *may* have factored in to the new supersized me. It had seemed like a good idea at the time.

I learned that it is actually very common for women, particularly those being treated for certain types of cancer, including breast cancer, to gain a significant amount of weight while undergoing chemotherapy. Ten to 15 pounds, some say. Great time for me to finally excel at something.

As I walked through the cancer centre on my chemo days, I began to see the similarities between myself and other women in the chemo suite. There really was a certain "chemo look" about us. The puffiness was all part of the treatment. The dark circles under my eyes– no doubt strong indicators of my extreme fatigue as my body fought to rebuild healthy cells that were constantly being destroyed chemically– were all part of the treatment. The depression, although present and actively being treated for years before my cancer diagnosis, was also a common side effect of the treatment. Good times all around.

I decided, after viewing some digital pictures that Monica had sent me of Claudia's baptism, that maybe I should cut down to one poutine a day and include some fruits and veggies in my diet. It sounds drastic, I know, but I was getting jollier by the minute. Pity party: officially over. Operation "I just want to be able to wear my big pants again": on.

Chapter 43:
My Visit to
Brant Avenue Public School

La Visite de Madame Nolan

Suddenly leaving work the way I did, literally working one day and not returning the next, was difficult. Dr. Fraser had written me a note on Friday. I was not to return to work on Monday. That was it. I was done. At the time, I was stopping work because of the painful varicose veins that were taking over both legs, partially as a result of being a big, pregnant woman on her feet all day long. Little did I know that the veins were only the beginning of my problems!

I stayed away from work for a very long time. Longer than I meant to. The longer I stayed away, the harder it was to return. I taught French as a Second Language to our junior students, in Grades 4 through 6. I taught a lot of kids! While normally very comfortable in my role as teacher, I felt like a cancer patient more than anything else in the early days.

Perhaps I didn't realize or admit it to myself right away, but my biggest fear about returning to work for a visit was actually facing the children. They would see Madame Nolan with a golden silk scarf around her head. Not much in the way of eyebrows or eyelashes. A very round face, puffy from the chemotherapy drugs. And I knew they would find a way to ask about it. I also knew that I could never bring myself to tell my students anything other than the complete truth.

The fact that I had left them all so suddenly had likely been explained in terms of my being pregnant. It was an easy assumption for children to make; I had left early to have my baby. Teachers came and went all the time; maternity leaves were commonplace at a school with so many young female teachers.

Eventually, I worked up the courage to face my fear. I bundled up Dana in her cutest pink girlie outfit (I had made the mistake, after having Bryn, of taking her to school in a blue and white outfit. I explained that "his" name was, in fact, Bryn and that Bryn was, in fact, a girl, more times than I care to remember. What was I thinking? Of course pink means girl and blue means boy. Duh!). I loaded her into her car seat, stroller in the trunk, purse in front seat. Off we went to Brant Ave. P.S.

It felt eerie entering the school. I was a visitor in my own workplace. I stopped by the office to say hello to Bruce Davies, the principal. We had a good visit and then Dana decided for me that it was time to get moving. I pushed the stroller onward, stopping briefly in the library to say hello to a few teachers and students that were there. It was almost recess time, and I figured I'd stay in the library until the bell rang and the kids all came running out of their classrooms to get ready to go outside. Dana, being on the fragile side at the best of times, might not have taken too kindly to being mobbed by screaming children immediately following the noise of a very loud recess bell.

The bell rang and out came the familiar faces of boys and girls I had not seen for many months. I still pictured them in last year's grades with last year's homeroom teachers. Funny how all change stops in the mind's eye when we are away from people for a while. Of course the kids had grown and changed. Yet, it made part of me a bit sad to see what I had missed. The other part was glad to have had a break, I admit it. Still, it felt good as some of my students noticed me, called out to me and came running to the library to meet Dana and give me hugs. Dana was spoiled rotten with all the attention she received and I soaked up the time with the kids.

As was inevitable, not long after our initial hugs and hellos, Courtnee, clearly the spokesperson of the group that day, asked me why I hadn't returned to Brant yet. I thought for a moment and then told her that I was still on maternity leave. I would be home with Dana for the entire school year. That was true, right? But kids are not stupid, and I knew we were not done talking about it yet.

Without skipping a beat, Courtnee and Jordan responded together that yes, I had had a baby, but that didn't explain why I hadn't returned yet. "Lots of teachers have babies but they come back. Why haven't you?" As I looked into their eyes and listened to them speak, it dawned on me that word of my cancer had already spread. They *knew*. They *all* knew. They wanted to see if I would tell them the truth. So I did.

I explained, feeling the blood rush to my cheeks from the discomfort of the situation, that I had been diagnosed with breast cancer while I was pregnant with Dana. I had had the cancer removed surgically and the doctors felt confident that they had gotten it all. Just to be safe, I was in the middle of chemotherapy treatments. That was why my hair was gone and I was wearing my bright headscarf. I was feeling great now, tired but happy, I assured them. It was fun being home with Dana and Bryn. Life was good. I was still Madame Nolan, the corny French teacher with the corny French music and games!

Thankfully, the truth was enough. They took it in bravely. They asked good questions and I answered them as best I could. They asked to see and touch my bald head. I felt okay with that, but didn't have the nerve to leave my headscarf off for very long.

Just a quick peek. But I did give them that. Then, very quickly, our talk turned to them. Clearly satisfied with what I had told them, it was so not about me anymore. They had stories about their new teachers, their friends, their families and so much more. They spoke quickly, loudly, each one trying to outtalk the other. As the bell rang, signalling that it was time for the kids to head back to class, I felt I had never left.

With the initial meeting over, I relaxed significantly and had the courage to walk into the junior hallway where the kids were hanging up their outdoor clothes and putting on their indoor shoes. I watched as more and more of my former students noticed me, nudged their friends, stared a bit and then finally smiled and waved. I waved back, saying "Bonjour" to several kids as they passed. I received many hugs and listened as children begged me to come back. By all accounts, they were having a good year with the teacher who had replaced me, but it felt really good to know that I had not been completely replaced in their hearts.

Chapter 44:
Bryn's Reaction to a Bald Mommy

One of these moms is not like the others

After the initial shock of seeing me without hair, Bryn became quite used to my new look. We had matching hats to wear and enjoyed wearing them around the neighbourhood for all to see. It was a mother-daughter thing.

At night, while I snuggled with Bryn in her bed (a habit I got into as much for my own comfort as for hers, and one that would prove very difficult to change later on), she would rub her hands across my smooth head and say "that feels funny" or "you lost your hair because of your cancer booboo medicine, right?". I reassured her when she brought it up, trying to be honest but not to focus too much on the cancer side of things.

One night, as we lay awake listing her friends by name (a favourite nightly ritual at that time), seemingly out of nowhere Bryn looked into my eyes and said, "I'm not going to lose my hair, right? I don't have a cancer booboo."

There have been so many moments throughout this experience that were unspeakably difficult, but none as devastating to my heart and soul as the ones involving my little girl. No mom wants her daughter to have to think about such serious, scary things. "Your beautiful hair will stay on your head forever, my love. You are just fine. Perfect." God, I pray you keep my children safe.

Later that same month, I took Bryn grocery shopping with me. While we were there, I decided we would buy a little gift for Bryn's friend, Benjamin, who was home sick with a terrible ear infection, one of many he'd had so far that winter. We went up and down the aisles, keeping an eye out for the perfect surprise get-well-soon treat.

At the end of one aisle we saw brightly coloured boxes. We took a closer look and found that inside the boxes were play plastic shaving kits. Perfect for Benjamin! He could play with the toys in his bathtub or shave alongside his dad in the mornings.

I let Bryn choose which set she'd like to give Benjamin (She picked Spiderman without hesitation). I rolled our cart up close enough for her to reach over and grab the box. No surprise when both arms found their way to the shelf, each hand grabbing a box. One for Benjamin. One for Bryn. I figured she could pretend to shave her legs in the tub. Why not?

Never have I seen Bryn more excited to take a bath than on that day. All day long she asked if it was bath time yet. I also suspect that she worked extra hard to get dirty (a gift that has always come naturally to her, not unlike Pigpen from the Charlie Brown cartoons) in the hopes of us having to give her a bath to keep her from ruining our entire house with her filth!

Finally, no later than 6 p.m. that evening, we caved and ran the water into the tub. In went the bubbles. Bryn tore open the box of shaving toys. All was well. She hopped in and I proceeded to scrub the grime of the day off her. Next, I washed her hair. All the while, she happily explored and experimented, thrilled with her new purchase.

I watched her play for a while, spraying pretend shaving foam on the tub ledge and delicately shaving it off again. Over and over and over and over. Good times. Have I mentioned that obsessive-compulsive disorders run in my family? You need only watch Bryn play for a short time to understand what I mean.

In any case, the game at last became a bore. Before I knew it, Bryn was dunking her head under the water, getting nicely soaked. She had never done that before. Then, to my surprise, she sprayed a massive amount of shaving cream into the palm of her hand and her hand went up to her hair. "What are you doing?" I asked. "I'm going to shave my head like you do", she replied with a grin.

Sure enough, she grabbed her plastic razor and methodically pretended to shave her hair off, one strip at a time. I am relatively certain that no other toddler in the neighbourhood was playing that particular tub game that night. Only at the Nolan house.

Chapter 45:
The Possibility of More Surgery

Hit me with your breast shot!

I was approximately midway through my chemotherapy treatments and had become quite comfortable with the whole "chemo thing". As with anything, after a while it had become a routine. None of us looked forward to it, but we didn't dread it anymore either. We just did it.

I walked into Dr. Tozer's office before my fourth or fifth chemo treatment. That was the way it always went on chemo days; first to the blood lab, then to Clinic D to talk to nurse Judy and Dr. Tozer about any problems or nasty side-effects that needed fixing, and then finally off to the chemo suite for my treatment.

I was feeling calm and relaxed. That should have been a huge sign that I was about to encounter a major bump in the road of my breast cancer journey. You know those signs that indicate a hidden road is up ahead? Without the sign, you would never see the road coming. That's what happened to me on this particular chemo day. Where did *that* road come from?

We discussed how I had been feeling over the three weeks since my last chemotherapy treatment. Quite well, actually. Very, very hungry. Very, very tired. Very, very achy on certain days. Other than that, not much to report. Dr. Tozer was pleased that it was going so well. I was handling the chemotherapy like a pro. Yes, I thought. I really was doing great. This chemotherapy thing wasn't so bad after all (yes it was, but at least I knew I could do it).

If this were a horror movie, you'd be hearing creepy music in the background right now indicating that a killer was behind me. "Run away!" you'd yell. But to no avail.

Soon, my dear oncologist reminded me, I would be going to my appointment to meet with the radiation oncologist, Dr. Sussman. Did I know that? Yes. He's the guy who would be telling me when I would begin my radiation treatments and how many I would be receiving, as well as how long each treatment would take. Right, doc? Not so much.

As it turned out, Dr. Tozer "strongly suspected" (which, I think, means "knew", but that's just me guessing) that at my meeting with Dr. Sussman, I would be told that radiation was not for me. Hooray! I didn't need radiation therapy! That was great news, given that I had heard how difficult such treatments can be on a person, especially closely following aggressive chemotherapy treatments.

Killer music getting louder.... "There's still time to run away! Go now!" Too late. I then learned the bad news. The reason I would not likely be a good candidate for radiation therapy was not because I didn't need it, but because my cancer had been multi-focal, not limited to one particular spot on my breast. And I was very young. Very, very young.

Radiation therapy, Dr. Tozer explained (and Dr. Sussman later confirmed), was best suited to treat a specific spot on the breast. In my case, it was impossible to find a perfect spot that would allow the radiation to get to all areas involved. Some microscopic cancer cells could be missed. Given my young age, the most aggressive treatment for me, the treatment that would give me the greatest chances of survival in the long run, was to have my right breast removed.

(Insert blood-curdling scream here.)

Chapter 46:
A Visit from Kate

The West Coast is in the house (er, Cancer Centre)!

There are people in this world who are all alone, without a single close friend with which to walk through life's ups and downs. I, on the other hand, have been blessed. Best friends, old and new, surround me.

Kate and I go way back. All the way back to Grade 8. She moved to London from Halifax, and she turned heads on the first day that she joined us in Mr. Goss' classroom. Not because of her beauty; at that time she was full of it, beauty I mean, but you had to dig deep.

She was tough. She was angry. And she had a presence that literally said, "Don't mess with me". I found her intriguing, frightening and endearing. I still can't say exactly what attracted me to her that day, but I was pulled to her and have been drawn to her time and time again ever since.

We became fast friends; a very unlikely pair. My friends didn't understand it, nor did hers. We were from different worlds, or so it would appear to everyone, even us, at times. Yet, when you peeled back the layers that each of us had grown around us, we were very much alike in many ways.

Kate had a heart of gold. Still does. She would do anything for anyone she loves. She doesn't let just anyone in to her world and her heart, but when she does, it is a gift. She is smart, funny, sarcastic and very courageous. I don't think she is able to see herself that way yet, but I'm working on it.

Kate had the guts to tell me she was a lesbian when we were still in high school. It mattered little to me, except that knowing made me feel like I knew *her* better. We were closer from the moment she told me and I was glad she had trusted me enough to tell me to my face.

Was it a great shock? Nope. I had often wondered if *she* knew she was a lesbian. Should I tell her she was? Haha. Her identity as a lesbian woman is only one part of who she is, but I believe it is a source of strength, pride and self-love. It makes her even better. It makes her more Kate.

Over the years, Kate and I have had our ups and downs. The highs were always very high, and some of the lows were nearly the end of us. Still, there is something, that "thing" that brought us together in the first place so long ago, that won't let us go our separate ways. We need each other and love each other too much.

It didn't come as a surprise that Kate flew from her current home, Vancouver, British Columbia, to stay with her dad in Oakville, Ontario while I was undergoing chemotherapy. She made a point to come and see me, to be with me and to give me strength through her love. As far as hospitals and medicine go, Kate's right up there with Jeff, competing for the title of "most likely to pass out". Still, she managed to put me before her terror and met me at the Juravinski Cancer Centre for one of my AC chemotherapy treatments.

I saw her walk through the front doors before she saw me. Her wavy hair blew in the breeze. Her face was solemn. Her nervousness was evident. I had never had to walk through those doors all alone. How did she do it that day? I waved at her through the window of the blood lab. I watched as relief flooded over her. She smiled that Kate smile and I knew we'd both be OK. We hugged, got teary, hugged some more. She took in my bald head for the first time (I had been nervous for her to see it) and touched it, amazed and I think a bit amused. She said I looked beautiful and at least part of me thinks she really meant it.

We went to Clinic D and waited for Dr. Tozer to call me in. We joked like old times, resorting comfortably to sarcasm to lighten the mood. My white blood cell count was good and I got the go-ahead to move up to the chemo suite. Again, routine for me, not so much for Kate.

That day I remember seeing the whole chemotherapy experience through Kate's eyes. I watched the chemo nurse seat us. I watched the needle go in. I watched the nurse push the red Adriamycin through the large tube into my arm. I watched the nurse hook up the Cyclophosphamide and get the drip going. I watched and listened as a dietitian came and spoke to me about healthy ways to eat during and after treatments (funny, no mention of poutine). I saw it all the way I'd see it if it were Kate in the chair and me by her side. I wanted nothing more than to run screaming the entire time.

When it was over, we headed for Guelph. Jeff drove while Shelley, Kate and I visited, sometimes talking a mile a minute, and other times not talking at all. At home, we told Jeff to have fun with the girls. We were off for a drink and a bite to eat. Mostly a drink. If Jeff was surprised to be ditched on chemo day, he didn't show it. He took one for the team.

Smitty's, while rarely the social meeting place of choice for those who are not yet eligible to receive a senior's discount, was close to home and all we had the energy for. They served cold drinks and appetizers, and we would provide our own entertainment. I can't remember what I ordered to drink. Nothing alcoholic, I'm guessing, what with the chemo and all.

Then again, stranger things have happened, and my notes indicate, in Tanya's bold printing, that some wine while on chemo is *OK*. Judy said so.

Kate and Shelley ordered nice cold drinks and we decided to share an order (OK, two) of onion rings. What was it the dietitian had said about eating well during chemo? Something about lots of fruits and veggies. Last time I checked, onions were veggies. Enough said.

We sat out on the patio and it was a beautiful sunny day. We all commented on the great weather. Yes, good times. Then we waited to see who would complain first about the sun in our eyes and the bees flying all around us.

Inside the restaurant, we got caught up on each other's lives. Lots had happened, and having a long-distance friendship is tough. It's so hard to keep up with the little things, the details of life that make it interesting. We did our best to fill each other in and enjoyed just being there in the moment. At one point, I asked Kate if I could have a sip of her drink. She didn't like it and was going to let it go to waste. We couldn't have that.

As I leaned in to take a sip from her straw, she pulled the drink away and, teasing me, said, "I can't catch your cancer, can I?" Of course she was kidding as only Kate could get away with, and let me take a sip, but it was one of those moments you never forget. Not because it upset me. I know Kate well enough to get her sense of humour, but because it made me realize that no matter how normal we pretended our visit was, the big pink elephant was still in the room. Cancer. At that time in my life, it never completely disappeared.

Chapter 47:
The Truth about Being Bald

Hats off to you

I say that I had become quite comfortable with my baldness, but perhaps I should clarify. There were times when I felt gorgeous. Just being alive made me feel beautiful. I was handling a difficult situation very well and to be honest, I was often proud of myself for that. So, yes, often I was comfortable with my shiny, hair-free head. Talk about wash and go.

However, the other side of my reality was that, as comfortable as I thought I was just letting my bald head show, I still felt the need to protect others from it. When I had plans with friends and family, I usually panicked if I couldn't find my head wrap immediately. I would put on my shiny, gold headpiece and then breathe a little easier.

I wanted to make others more comfortable with me. It felt like making people look at my bald head was forcing them to think about my cancer. That was the last thing I wanted. I wanted to blend in; to be just one in a crowd. Just Marcie. Not Cancer Marcie.

This baldness/comfort issue brings me to my gals. I have yet to talk about my closest circle of friends here in Guelph, the Baby Basics Group. When I first had Bryn, I was relatively new to Guelph and had no close friends in the city outside of my work colleagues. Upon leaving the hospital to start my new life as a mother, I was handed a folder full of pamphlets, important phone numbers and information to read at home.

One day I flipped through the folder while Bryn, then colicky in a way you could never be prepared for even if you tried, exercised her obviously very healthy lungs. She was quite newly born and already the walls of our tiny downtown apartment were starting to close in around me. I had to get out, but where could I go?

I came upon an information sheet about a group called Baby Basics. It was a free six-week program offered to new mothers by the public health nurses. There were two locations to choose from. There was a number to call and a contact name. To register, you simply had to call and say you wanted to be a part of the group. That easy. If it had been any more complicated than that, I honestly believe I would not have had the energy to even bother. Thankfully, it is a group for brand new moms, so whoever set it up knew the state most new moms are in!

I received confirmation of my registration and arrived early to our very first meeting. Around a circle sat a group of tired new moms, all seemingly in my age group. All with wrinkled little people. All with bags under their eyes (the moms, that is). All with baby vomit somewhere on their clothes. All obviously happy to be out of the house and in adult company for a change.

From literally the very first BB meeting, I felt a part of something special. Slowly, over the six-week program, we got to know each other by name. Actually, most of us knew each other as "Benjamin's mom" or "Julia's mom" for a long time, and then slowly it became as much about us as our babies.

When the final meeting was coming to an end, I felt that I had met several women I could relate to on various levels. I hated the idea of walking away, going back to my apartment and back to being alone (with an angry baby). I gathered up my courage and raised my hand. I asked if anyone would be interested in signing her name and phone number on a sheet and continuing to meet once a week, informally, taking turns at each other's houses. I admit that the teacher in me had emerged the night before, and I had typed out an official-looking page with spaces for names, phone numbers, addresses and e-mail addresses. Some things never change. I hoped that we could remain friends.

To my relief, everyone signed the sheet and seemed happy to continue the friendships that had only just begun to blossom. It has now been more than six years since our group first met and many new children have been born, joining the fun. Only a couple of people have drifted, outgrowing their need for the group. The rest of us are in it for the long haul.

We have enjoyed house parties, park trips, hiking excursions, picnics and more. The best part is, of course, that we all became confident, loving mothers who are not afraid to leave our kids at home for some "daddy time". Now, more often than not, we have "mom's night out" dinners. It's no longer solely about the babies. We do share stories about our angels from time to time, but we have way more to talk about than our children alone. True friendships have formed that go beyond the trials and tribulations of new mommy hood.

This brings me back to my original point. It is this group of friends that I wanted so much to protect from my obvious baldness. I imagined them looking at my head and being unable to see past it, past the cancer treatments. Of course, I should have known them better. It was definitely my own insecurity that led me to cover up in my friends' presence.

Throughout my treatments, I joined in on lots of fun times with the BB ladies. Each time, I donned my sparkling wrap, put on some cheek colour and lip gloss and attempted to look as bright and healthy as I possibly could. Just blend in.

I haven't mentioned Julie yet, but she was one of my biggest supports through thick and thin. Julie and I have some things in common, including our need for "me time" and our preference to spend time with one or the other of our children as opposed to both at once. We also both have the guts to admit that out loud. Oh, and we *love* food. Big time. Julie is one of the ones who fed us regularly all through my chemo treatments. Many other moms in the group also spoiled us regularly, dropping by with casseroles, desserts, flowers, you name it.

Julie is the mom in the group that we can always count on to be brutally honest. She's not afraid to tell it like it is and it's one of the things I love (and fear) most about her. We all do, I think.

I am far too worried about what others think, always have been, to openly and easily speak my mind. I admit to having an internal filter constantly working in my head, processing through what I should or shouldn't say. Julie, it seems, has no such filter.

It is only fitting, then, that it was Julie who eventually spoke the truth about my baldness, or my attempts to "blend in" by use of a wrap. She let me know that it was way creepier for everyone to see me in my "chemo wrap" than to simply see me bald.

It's not like they saw my covered head and thought to themselves, "Oh good, Marcie's not on chemo. She can't be. She's not bald." In fact, Julie pointed out, they all felt very comfortable with my bald head, much more so than the hat look.

It turns out that the look I was most comfortable with myself, bald and beautiful, was also the look that made my friends most comfortable. They could get used to the hairless me easily and after visiting for a few minutes could largely forget about it. It was just me, just Marcie, the way I wanted to be seen. As soon as I put on the wrap, it was like a neon sign, saying "Cancer. Cancer. Cancer". Far more difficult to see past that.

I absolutely understand what Julie meant and thank God for a true, honest, loving friend who cares enough and trusts our friendship enough to put it all out there.

Chapter 48:
More Help from the BB Moms

A casserole a day keeps the cancer away

While Julie was the one in the mom's group who always spoke the truth, however good or bad it may have been, there were so many others who also reached out to us as my cancer experience unraveled before us.

It began with me e-mailing Liz Luhta and telling her about my diagnosis. I would have called her to talk about it, as we had become quite close since our first meeting almost three years ago, but I was not able to speak the truth to her out loud. Not yet. So, I asked Liz if she would mind e-mailing the rest of the group to let them know that I had cancer and would be having a lumpectomy in May. She sent an e-mail immediately. It was perfect. It was compassionate, sympathetic and said everything I wanted my friends to know.

Once the word was out, the flowers started arriving by the dozen. Gorgeous, bright bouquets from my friends. Cards of support and love that made me cry every time I read them. Each time the phone rang, it turned out to be another florist wanting to deliver more flowers for me, for us. I placed the multi-coloured gifts in vases all over my main floor. Just looking at them and smelling them in the air made me feel better. A bit calmer. I needed that.

Next, the best part of all: food. Deliveries of food from everyone! Laura-Lee McKeown dropped off a homemade chicken pot pie and a delicious strawberry cream dessert. It was gone the same night we received it! She also brought cute matching outfits for my girls.

Lori Payne, a beautiful kind soul in our group, brought my family an amazing home-cooked meal to eat on the night of my surgery. I would be fed in the hospital, and she knew they would be in no shape to cook. She delivered the meal, complete with oven gloves and salad tongs. She left out nothing. My family later raved about Lori and her kindness. Her meal was tasty and her thoughtful gesture to them (and me) much appreciated.

Liz, after delivering my news to the gals, prepared for me what has become one of my absolute favourite comfort foods. It is a creamy, cheesy chicken and pasta vegetable casserole. It is basically the perfect combination of all things comforting and yummy. It is a huge casserole, enough to feed us all a few times. It just gets better and better every time we taste it! To this day, Bryn requests "Liz's supper". I have yet to try to re-create it in my own kitchen. My fear is that it will fall short of the one made with Liz's loving hands.

I recall that on the night before my family and I drove to Hamilton to meet the cancer team for the first time, Trish Goodridge arrived at the door with hugs and the most unbelievable vegetarian lasagna I've ever tasted! Again, it was huge and comforting: perfect for that time in my life. I thanked Trish and put it in the fridge to have the next night for dinner. I knew that my family and Jeff's would be at our house discussing all that we had heard and learned at Juravinski, and the lasagna would be enough to feed us all, and then some.

Sure enough, as we arrived home from Hamilton, our heads spinning with an overload of information, her fresh lasagna was the perfect meal. We sat around the table eating (even *I* ate some and my appetite had been as good as gone since my diagnosis), talking, and just allowing our bodies to be filled back up. We'd all need the energy to get through the events to come.

Monica Peirson-Durbin prepared us a full dinner. A feast fit for a king. At least she tells me it was fit for a king. As it turned out, I went out of town to London for a few days with little notice, and Monica had prepared a fresh meal for me assuming I'd be home. I did not get back in time to receive her meal, and it couldn't go to waste, so Monica, Dave, Benjamin and Claudia ate it in our honour. It still counts as a special meal made with love for us and we enjoyed hearing about it. If Monica ever finds herself in a situation where she could use help with a meal, I'll be happy to make and eat one for her anytime!

Tammy Watson, the mother of all mothers and friends, went into "caregiver" mode immediately upon receiving Liz's e-mail and brought us full dinners, complete with all food groups, at least 10 times. On "Tammy nights", my family saw how other families live. How other mothers cook. How other people eat. I knew that at some point, when I was well again, I'd be back on my own to do the cooking, and it occurred to me that Tammy had raised the bar much higher than it had been! We enjoyed each savoury morsel, gratitude filling us up as much as the meals themselves.

I'm sure you can imagine that, with all the food pouring in from friends, neighbours and family, we ended up buying a large freezer for our basement. It is human nature, it seems, that when people feel powerless to change a situation they prepare food as an offering to the suffering body and soul. It *is* just what the doctor ordered, for anyone in any crisis.

Chapter 49:
The Decision to
Remove My Right Breast

Is the bra half empty or half full?

A complete mastectomy, the surgery in which the entire breast is removed, had crossed my mind more than once. Soon after my cancer diagnosis, I emotionally distanced myself, to a large degree, from my affected breast. The breast had inevitably come to represent cancer. It would never again be the same lovely, B-cupped body part that I (and Jeff) had known and loved for what seemed like forever. Impossible. So, the idea of having my right breast removed entered my brain early on in this process.

Another reason that I toyed with the mastectomy option early on was my fear of dying. It's that simple. The more I thought about the cancer that had invaded my right breast, the more I wanted to take the most aggressive route possible to kick the disease's butt. Hard. If removing my breast would buy me even one more hour on earth with my loved ones, then bring it on.

I'm not making light of the issue, I assure you. No one, especially a young woman with dreams of a long and fulfilling future, wants to lose a part of herself. A part of herself that is so intimately linked to her femininity, her identity as a female. Her "womanness".

Plus, we all know how sexualized the female breast has become in our society. If breasts make me beautiful or sexy to the world, what will a mastectomy make me? My body image has greatly improved over the years, but could it withstand the amputation of a breast? Easy to say "sure" in theory, but in practice?

The other factor that I considered deeply when thinking about life without a breast was the possibility of life without breast pain. My recovery from the lumpectomy had been extremely painful every moment of every day. I have met many women who have also undergone a lumpectomy, and none seems to have experienced the degree or duration of pain that I did.

It could certainly have much to do with the fact that I was 7-1/2 months pregnant at the time. I was unable to take much in the way of pain relieving medication. I took Tylenol 3s in the early days following the surgery, but was soon enough on my own to feel the pain in all its fury. The breasts tend to be sore enough on a good day while a woman is pregnant, so to go ahead and mess with them further did nothing but fuel the fire.

The idea of removing my breast completely made me wonder if no breast would eventually hurt less than one that had been tampered with. It may sound odd, but the pain was so intense that many times I wished the breast would just disappear entirely. As each day went by and the pain continued to show no signs of letting up, I more and more often found my mind wandering to the possibility of a breast-less existence.

Finally, I seriously considered the removal of my right breast early on in the process because I had come to believe that as long as the breast was still attached to the rest of me, then there would always be a possibility that some cancer had been missed. The chances seemed much greater that the original cancer, if missed, would manage to make its way out of the breast and into body parts that I really couldn't live without. So the lumps had been successfully removed as well as the DCIS, but in my mind, at least, the cancer still had a place to call home if it chose to return.

Chapter 50:
Genetic Testing Options

Ripped genes

My family has been riddled with cancer. For as long as I can remember, everyone who has died on my mother's side of the family has died of one form of cancer or another (with the exception of my own mother who died so young that I will never know if she would have developed cancer had she lived past the age of 49). While a variety of cancers are somewhat common in our family line, it is definitely breast and prostate cancers that win the gold medal.

On my mom's side, my grandpa, Lawrence Forestell, died of prostate cancer. He had five sisters. Every one of them died of breast cancer before they reached menopause. One was only 29 years old. Growing up aware of our family's history with cancer, especially breast cancer in women and prostate cancer in men, my cousins, sister and I had an awareness of the disease that, while not at the forefront of our minds at all times, I believe lurked in the background for years, scaring us and threatening our happiness and good health.

Looking at the next generation, my mom's generation, did nothing to assuage our fears. My mom's sister, Dianne Yates, fought long and hard to beat breast cancer when she was only beginning menopause. My Aunt Dianne had felt for a long time that something was not right and had seen a number of doctors, all of whom told her that her breast was fine. Very soon after my mom died, Aunt Dianne felt a sharp pain in her breast and knew for certain that something was terribly wrong. Later, she described the feeling she had had that my mother was with her, warning her. The pain, she believed, was my mother's way of getting her back to the doctor and of encouraging her to make them take her seriously. Pain is not generally a symptom of breast cancer (my own tumour caused no pain at all), so in my mind, it is absolutely possible that Dianne was right about my mom. I choose to believe her.

Finally, my aunt was given the diagnosis we had all feared: breast cancer. By the time her cancer was discovered, it had had time to metastasize to other parts and was slowly taking over. I remember how courageously she endured her chemo, treatment after treatment. She lost her hair but continued to be absolutely beautiful. I still lived in London at that time, as did she, so I got to spend a lot of time with her while she was on her breast cancer journey.

Dianne worked at the University of Western Ontario, the university I attended. Often, we met for lunch or when she was finished work for the day. We'd sit and have a bite to eat and talk about all kinds of things. She was easy to talk to and had taken me under her wing after my mom died. I knew I could always talk to her about anything at all. And I did.

One image of my aunt that has remained firmly in my mind is of her during one of our university visits. We had gone to the bathroom and were washing our hands. Dianne was very nearly bald, with only tiny spikes of hair, but she took a bright red lipstick from her purse and leaned in to the mirror to apply it to her lips. I watched her closely and wondered at that moment what she thought when she looked at herself. She seemed so confident, so content. It blew my mind that this woman I was standing with had cancer. It was impossible.

As courageous as she was, once the cancer beast got out of its cage, Dianne could not outrun it forever. Her treatments and participation in many clinical trials, her willingness to be a guinea pig to advance research and hopefully benefit from new advancements that were being tested, eventually wore her out. The cancer had invaded her bones and her liver.

When there were no more treatment options left for her, when her care became palliative in nature, the pain she experienced was immense. Her husband, Dave, her daughter, Jen, and her son, Pat, were with her at her home when she died. That was where she had wanted to be in her final moments. Losing Aunt Dianne to breast cancer changed me. I have never been the same or felt the same since. It confirmed that none of us was safe.

Having been through my own journey and looking back, there are so many things I understand that I didn't understand back then. There are so many things I'd do differently if I could go back. I would have asked Dianne more about how she was coping. I'd have talked to her about how she felt, not just physically but emotionally. I would not have so easily accepted her cheerful assurances that she was doing great, even when I knew she couldn't have been. I know now that she was protecting me. I hate myself for letting her.

I would not have hidden behind deep denial, ignoring the obvious, never bringing up the fact that she had cancer. And it was spreading. I would have really *been there* for her. I would have put my own fears aside and asked her how I could help; what I could do. I still think about her often and pray that she knew how much I loved her. I think she did.

The next to be attacked by the insidious disease was my gentle, soft-spoken Uncle Gerry, Lawrence's son. He had been unwell for quite some time but kept it to himself. He was never one to go to the doctor, nor was he one to bother others with his problems. No one in our family really knew just how ill he was right up until he died. There had been talk that he looked thin. People had shared their theories and fears about what might be wrong but no one knew he was dying. I didn't, at least. He had wanted it that way.

By the time Uncle Gerry did seek medical attention, his prostate cancer had run rampant. He grew thinner and thinner and, in the end, became the next victim of cancer in our family. I can still picture him, his quiet, loving spirit. I never had long conversations with him over the years, but I always felt comfortable in his presence. He was the uncle I could just sit beside and not feel as if I needed to talk for the sake of filling the quiet around us.

He was also one of the only people to respond immediately to my request, soon after my mom died, for pictures of and stories about my mom. I had wanted, needed, to know who my mom was to the people in her life. Gerry pulled me aside at a family function once and told me how he had so many wonderful memories and stories about Nancy. The twinkle in his eyes as he spoke about her was worth more to me than any picture he could have handed me. Now I have the memory of him, that day, smiling at me so genuinely and I hold it dear. Always will.

My uncle Jack, Lawrence's other son, was treated for prostate cancer, too. He had gone to his doctor for a completely different reason when his cancer was detected. Thankfully his cancer was in the very early stages and was easily treatable. He underwent radiation therapy and was declared cancer-free.

For about five years, Uncle Jack fought a winning battle with prostate cancer. Then, unbelievably, he was dealt another mighty blow: he had lung cancer. Jack's lung cancer was not the result of his prostate cancer metastasizing. It was a new primary cancer. Our family could *not* seem to get a freaking break. Seriously.

Jack bravely made regular trips to Hamilton from Guelph (he, too, was being treated at the Juravinski Cancer Centre) to undergo radiation and chemotherapy treatments. One day when I was at Juravinski for my chemotherapy, Shell and I were walking to the cafeteria when we ran into Uncle Jack. He was there for radiation in an attempt to shrink the tumour on his lung. Only in our family could people just run into each other accidentally at a cancer centre!

Sadly, the lung cancer, while kept at bay for quite a long period of time, did eventually spread to Uncle Jack's brain, ultimately ending his battle with cancer and his life. He meant so much more, touched so many more lives, than I could ever adequately write about here.

Perhaps the most devastating news our family has had to come to terms with involves my cousin Anne-Marie, Jack's oldest daughter, her husband, Sonny, and the eldest of their two beautiful daughters. Samantha, only 11 years old at the time, began complaining to her mother that she was extremely tired. She had no energy and was uninterested in playing with her friends. One Saturday night, she even decided against attending a slumber party. That was not at all like Sam, the social, friendly little girl that Anne-Marie and Sonny knew.

Anne-Marie decided to take Samantha to the doctor, thinking she must have been coming down with the flu or a bug of some kind. The nurse took blood to do some tests and the results were (and still are to this day) incomprehensible. Samantha needed to be taken immediately, from the doctor's office in Guelph, to the Children's Hospital in Hamilton. Her blood did not look right. Something was terribly, terribly wrong.

There they received news that no mother or father (or little sister, Ali) should ever have to hear: Samantha had leukemia. Leukemia, a cancer of the blood cells, does not seem to be hereditary, so why was ours, of all families, forced to deal with such a random, vicious disease? Samantha spent most of the rest of her life in the hospital, returning home for visits from time to time in the early days. She underwent gruelling chemotherapy treatments and was devastated as she lost her beautiful, long, black hair. The thought of that wonderful little girl so bravely accepting her diagnosis brings tears to my eyes.

Once, when Anne-Marie and Sonny sat down to tell their daughter that her blood problem had turned out to be a disease called leukemia, Samantha looked up at her parents and said that she knew what leukemia was and that she'd had a dream once that she would die of a disease by that name. Did she know on some level that this would be her fate? I believe she did.

When Samantha died at age 11, it was like a light of hope went out in all of us. If it was possible for such a cruel, devastating thing to happen to a little girl, then what hope was there for the rest of us? It didn't make sense and it made me angry. Very angry. I'm sure I'm not the only one who questioned God, demanding an explanation. Why *her*? Why not one of *us*? Samantha had brightened up the world in her short life. Her future was stolen from her, and we will all miss out on so much because of it.

Needless to say, I have always been pretty certain that something genetic was predisposing us to cancer. I had no proof, but knew in my gut that the number of cancers in our family was more than a fluke. Some of us have even grown up thinking of cancer more in terms of "when" than "if" we got it.

Being diagnosed with my most feared disease at only 32 years of age got us all thinking, yet again, about our family history and genetic history. Perhaps the gene pool was a bit murky? Good thing the Forestell sense of humour and love of beer were also being passed down, as we all needed lots of both to endure diagnosis after diagnosis and death after death.

Sometime before I began my own chemotherapy treatments, I was offered the opportunity to participate in a genetic test that I was told might determine if I was born predisposed to breast cancer. Given that I was absolutely sure that cancer ran in my family by way of genes, I was anxious to know if my girls and my sister (and all of my relatives on mom's side) were at a much greater risk for cancer themselves.

Recent genetic research has clearly demonstrated that there are at least two genetic mutations specifically linked to an increased risk of breast and ovarian cancers. These genetic mutations are known as BRCA 1 and BRCA 2 (Breast Cancer 1 and 2). Over time, as dedicated researchers continue to study genetics, more links may be found and more mutations may be isolated. For now, there are two mutations you don't want to have, BRCA 1 and BRCA 2.

There was very little discussion between Jeff, myself and my immediate family before I opted to participate in the testing. It wasn't 100 percent accurate; in fact, the testing is still very new and has a high incidence of false positives. Sometimes the test results are simply inconclusive and you leave knowing nothing more than you did before the test. Still, I wanted to try.

The genetic test itself, from a patient standpoint, was very simple. I went to Juravinski Cancer Centre, headed for the blood lab, closed my eyes and waited for the needle. A handful of vials of blood later, no more than three or four, if memory serves me, and I was on my way home. My part was done and the rest was up to science.

I had been counselled intensely before actually making my final decision. The details had been explained and I understood as much as I was ever going to. By the genetic counsellor's estimation, based on my family history of cancer and my age at cancer diagnosis, there was somewhere around a 20 to 25 per cent chance that I would test positive for a BRCA mutation. Not *that* great a chance.

The genetic counsellor had specifically warned us that the testing was very intricate and took a great deal of time to complete. We were looking at a wait of three to four months before the results would be available. I drove home from the centre and felt relieved that at least I was actively trying to determine what was up with my family history and, thankfully, the mutations were extremely rare and it was not terribly likely that I would end up having either one. I'm sure everything would turn out just fine. Right....

Chapter 51:
My Decision to Remove Both Breasts

Do you offer a two-for-one deal?

Initially I had told my oncologist that I wanted my right breast removed. This was right after my diagnosis. I'll admit, I was probably hysterical at the time, but still, I put it out there. At that time, Dr. Tozer assured me that such a surgery would not likely be necessary. We let that issue rest for the time being. There was enough to worry about already.

So, much later on, as I listened to Dr. Sussman, the radiation oncologist, explain in great detail, and with an impeccable bedside manner, why a mastectomy was by far the best option for me, I was confident that my gut feeling way back when had been correct. It was a mastectomy I needed and it was a mastectomy I would have. Dr. Tozer, as always, was extremely supportive of this decision and helped me navigate through the details of what was to come.

Only I had two breasts to consider. I was very young, as everyone kept reminding me. I had a wicked family history of breast cancer. I could remove the right breast, but what about the left? If I was prone to breast cancer, did it make sense to tempt fate by assuming the left breast would remain cancer-free? Was it foolish to remove a perfectly healthy breast in a desperate attempt to prevent a possible future tumour?

I thought long and hard about the impact my cancer experience had had on my daughters. It was Bryn that I worried about the most. Dana was very young, happy to be held, fed and bathed by any family member or close friend that we entrusted her to. Bryn, on the other hand, understood some of what was happening. She has always been a serious girl who doesn't miss a thing. Explaining the removal of a breast to her was a conversation I couldn't fathom having.

Yet, the idea of having one breast removed first, only to be followed some time later with the removal of the other breast in the event of a new cancer, seemed more disruptive to our family life and routine. Wouldn't it be better to just be done with the surgeries all at once? Besides, I figured, it's not like saving one breast wouldn't be creepy. How much creepier would removing both be? The thought of being lopsided, for me, was worse than the idea of being flat but symmetrical.

It is a very personal decision that every woman must make for herself. There is no right way or wrong way to proceed. No one can tell you what is best for you. Family and friends may share their views, thoughts and opinions (sometimes even when you don't ask for their advice), but in the end, each woman makes the decision alone. After much thoughtful deliberation and many, many sleepless nights, I decided to do what had felt right, deep down in my gut, all along.

Chapter 52:
A New Chemotherapy Treatment

A kinder, gentler poison

My chemotherapy treatments continued, every third Friday, throughout the fall and into the winter. When I completed my fourth treatment, I was feeling extremely comfortable with how it worked. I knew on which days I would have an upset stomach, constipation (too much information?), mouth sores and achy muscles. I swear, it was like clockwork.

How was it that on the first Tuesday after each treatment, it was time for my entire body to feel as though it had been run over by a Mac truck and just barely survived? How, by Wednesday night, did I feel as though the pain of Tuesday had never really happened? How did my body respond the exact same way, all four treatments, without fail? This was very helpful to me, as I am a person who needs routine to feel comfortable. I had slipped into a routine that made the entire process much easier to bear. On a bad pain day, I could tell myself that it would all be better by the next evening. And it would be. Amazing.

My comfortable routine came to a grinding halt on chemotherapy treatment number five. I was done my four treatments of Adriamycin and Cyclophosphamide, thank God. However, I was now looking at a whole new drug, called Taxol, and didn't know what to expect. I felt initially as though I were starting chemotherapy all over again. I was nervous, couldn't eat (a rare thing for me, especially since starting the steroids) and dreaded the drive to Hamilton. Nurse Judy had told me that Taxol was a completely different drug with many different side effects. Everyone reacts differently, and some women even found Taxol much easier to tolerate, less taxing on their systems, than the AC.

Taxol, I learned, is a plant-based drug (I believe it comes from the bark of trees in some far away place, but I could be wrong). The good news was that some women's hair started coming back while on this drug. Please be me, please be me, please be me. The bad news was that a) it was often the cause of severe muscle and joint pain, b) some people did find it a more difficult drug to tolerate and, most importantly to me, c) unlike the AC treatments that only took about an hour to inject, the Taxol was a long, slow process.

Due to the fact that it is plant based, the chemotherapy nurses (amazing, amazing people at Juravinski, by the way) had to monitor patients very closely for allergic reactions to it. I would be given lots of Benadryl by IV and would wait for it to kick in. Then the Taxol would begin, and the nurses would watch me like a hawk in the early moments of my first injection. A severe allergic reaction would happen instantly, after the very first drop of Taxol entered my bloodstream. That quickly. Most people don't suffer from an allergic reaction, but they had no way of knowing who would be affected until they injected it. Well, my luck had been great thus far, so I was confident I'd be fine. Haha.

Chapter 53:
Taxol Treatment #1

We all need a Pink Lady

When I was sitting in the chemotherapy suite waiting area on the Friday of my first Taxol treatment, a worried woman caught my eye. Was it her very first time at the chemo suite? That's a feeling you never forget. She smiled brightly at me, her face beautiful, and introduced herself as Sandy. Her partner, a quiet, gentle man, was Paul. From the moment I met them, I could see that they were a strong team, working together to get through something huge and horrible. I could relate. So could Jeff. We liked them instantly.

Sandy mentioned that I looked great bald, which was my regular state at the Cancer Centre (at Juravinski you stand out if you *have* hair, not the other way around!). She confirmed my original thought. It *was* her very first day of chemotherapy and she was scared. She wanted to know how bad it really was. I did my best to comfort her, telling her that so far, it hadn't really been unbearable. Crappy, but do-able.

Sandy was able to talk to me candidly, honestly, about her journey. She had been travelling, doing outdoorsy things and, up to that point, felt like a million bucks. At some point while hiking, she became aware of a bloating, upset stomach. Naturally, she figured it was from drinking the water or something she ate. When she returned home at the end of her trek, the bloating was much, much worse and she knew she needed to see a doctor. As you have likely guessed by now, it was not the water. It was not the food. It was ovarian cancer and it had spread. Even having been diagnosed with a form of cancer myself, I still cannot even fathom what Sandy felt upon hearing those words. I do know that her life was forever changed at that exact moment in time, never to return to what it once was.

As Sandy and I shared our stories, we bonded. In a way, we were both in the same boat as far as the Taxol went. I had never tried it yet and neither had she. The difference was that I was already bald from previous chemo treatments, and she had a gorgeous head of short, funky hair to lose. So, we prayed that we would get beds together.

For the injection of Taxol, patients are given beds to lie down on. The whole process, with the drug injected slowly to prevent allergic reactions and not overload the system, would take approximately three to five hours in total. Again, thank God for Oprah's book club! I'd have some time to read for sure.

I explained the crazy number system (or lack thereof) to my new friends and we crossed our fingers that we would somehow get in together. We decided that since I had number three and she had number 61, we were sure to be called together! I loved Sandy's openness and sense of humour, and Paul and Jeff were cut from the same cloth. I'm sure it was good for them to talk a bit (even if it was about the news, sports, anything but why we were all there), each man knowing he was not the only one in the world with a young wife with cancer.

In the long-standing tradition of bad luck for me, Sandy was called first and Jeff and I were left to wait. And wait. Until, much to our surprise, relief and delight, a chemo nurse called my name and led me straight to Sandy's bed. The bed next to hers was empty, and my nurse offered it to me. It turns out that Sandy had used her wit and charm to convince the chemo nurse that, even if it wasn't my turn yet, I should be able to at least lie there while I waited. The bed was free anyway, right? She wasn't asking anyone to start up my Taxol until my turn, but pleeeease give me a bed in the meantime. Man, she's good!

And so Sandy and I became Taxol buddies, together every third Friday. I looked forward to my time with her (and Paul) and it made chemo feel like more of a social gathering than medical treatment. We laughed, sometimes too loud, and ate like we were on a cruise. No loss of appetite for Sandy, either, I was happy to see!

Since that first Taxol experience, with Sandy by my side, we've been friends. I love to read her e-mails and can hear her talking as I read them. Her road with ovarian cancer continues to be a winding one, with some steep hills, but she is certainly up for the challenge. We were in it together from the start for a reason; we had both needed each other to lean on. We still do. I am so happy, looking back, that I was able to be Sandy's Pink Lady.

Chapter 54:
The Support of Our Church

A gift from God

God works in mysterious ways. In the year leading up to my cancer diagnosis, Jeff and I had been searching for a church to call our own. We were feeling disconnected from our current church and knew it was time to move on. But to what? To where?

For a long while we simply stopped attending church altogether. We had been feeling for so long that we would rush around on Sunday mornings to get ourselves and Bryn ready for church in order to arrive on time (not an easy feat, with a spirited child!) only to arrive feeling alone. We had attended the church for more than a year and had not made any friends. No one knew our names or made eye contact to greet us. We weren't attending church to make best friends, but we wanted to join a congregation and become a meaningful part of the church community.

As time passed, our Sunday mornings at home did not feel right. We missed church. We missed being a part of a church community. We missed the choir's songs. We missed the quiet time to pray in God's house. We missed our connection with God. Somehow, much as we were doing our best to live Christian lives and to teach Bryn our beliefs, we were like sheep that had lost our way. And we knew it.

We were at the point of discussing our options but had not made any real effort to find a new church. We knew what we were looking for but had never really put it into words for each other. Jeff had his thoughts and I had mine. Both of us knew it was a matter of time before we would indeed find the "right fit", whatever that would turn out to be for us as a family.

As luck (or God) would have it, when we were made proud godparents to Claudia Durbin we had attended her baptismal ceremony at the Dublin Street United Church. There we had met an amazing husband and wife team, Reverends Sue Campbell and John Lawson. Jeff and I immediately warmed to them, feeling at ease and a part of the experience, not as strangers but as welcomed visitors.

Sue and John had heard our story from Monica and Dave, regular members of the church for many years. So when we entered the church and were introduced to the reverends, it felt as though we had met before. This was partly because they already knew of us, but mostly because they are so accepting and warm.

After the baptism and celebration that followed at the Durbin house, Jeff and I drove home. We got into our car and immediately began talking about our experience that day, our impressions of Sue and John, and our feelings about the church and service (and there was lots of talk about our Claudia, too!). It didn't take long for us to realize that we were on the same page. Neither one of us could explain it exactly, but we had found what we were looking for. Our church.

Since that time we have become members of Dublin Street United Church and Dana was later baptized there. We felt that we had found the spiritual connection we were looking for and have enjoyed the support and close community of the reverends and members of the congregation. It is very reassuring to know that we have a spiritual community that we can look to for support when we need it, and to whom we can offer support as well.

Chapter 55:
The Days Leading Up to
My Bilateral Mastectomies

That took balls!

Once the decision was made to remove both breasts, I spoke to Dr. Tozer and Dr. MacGillivray. I was anxious to get on with it. My dream was to have all surgeries behind me once and for all. It didn't take long before Dr. MacGillivray, God love her, had booked my OR time once again. My surgery was set for January 24th, 2006 at ten o'clock in the morning. Knowing the exact date and time that I would lose my breasts was both comforting and disconcerting in equal measure.

By this time, it was November and everyone was counting down until Christmas holidays. In my case, it was even more exciting to look ahead to Christmas, given that my final chemotherapy treatment was scheduled for December 16th. I'd be all done by the holidays. Plus, my surgery was not until the end of January, so there was a long enough break from all medical concerns to really focus on friends, family and food.

One day, Erin and Max drove to our house so that the kids could make Christmas gift bags. I had gone mad at the dollar store, buying plain brown paper gift bags, paint, glue, feathers, glitter, stencils, stickers; all manner of festive-coloured supplies. Our young artists would be thrilled! I can't even describe how great it felt to be doing "normal" things like everyone else.

We covered the kitchen table with a huge plastic tablecloth. Then, we organized all of the art supplies. We got Bryn and Max into their art smocks and assigned seats. We had two of everything, so no one would have to share. We had thought of everything. Did I mention Erin and I are both teachers? No pressure, kids.

At last it was time to let the kids express themselves creatively through art. We were active, loving, supportive parents. We were proud moms. We were crazy. Within minutes there was glue on the floor, feathers stuck to the tablecloth and paint on both of Bryn's hands and up one arm. No signs of any decorated gift bags yet. Perhaps six large bags each was a bit much for a three and five year old to tackle?

Still, we pushed on. We hovered, handed the kids items we knew would look darling on the bags, if only they would use them. We suggested that the cotton balls, when glued, would look like snow. The feathers were red and green, Christmas colours. The sparkles would be catchy to the eye. Oh, wouldn't Grandma and Grandpa be surprised to see the fancy homemade bags?

Our merriment became more and more forced, and there was tension in the air. Erin and I were trying hard to keep it together in front of each other and the children. I wondered which one of us would be the first to snap and threaten her child that Santa wouldn't come if the gift bags weren't decorated appropriately? Who's kidding whom? It was the teachers in the room who wanted to have arts and crafts time. The kids just wanted to snuggle on the couch together and watch Dora. All this and we hadn't even started the homemade chocolate project yet. Ho ho ho.

On another occasion, Erin and I had planned for Max and Bryn to make gingerbread houses together. It was Max's first Christmas in Canada, his first Christmas with his family. It was also their first Christmas together as cousins and we wanted to create lasting memories to be passed down from generation to generation.

I had found ready-to-decorate houses while out shopping one day and, being delusional most of the time when it comes to my child's actual personality and interests (not to mention attention span), I had bought two. One for my gifted daughter. One for my gifted nephew. Again, no pressure.

Large garbage bags were spread out on the kitchen floor, creating a bright, spacious art environment for our Picassos. We mixed the icing and poured it into two bowls. We literally counted out every single candy decoration so each child would get the same number and a nice variety of colours. Then we let them at it.

By the time I handed Bryn her bowl of icing, she had eaten half of her candy decorations and was showing no signs of stopping. Max spread most of his icing on one side of his house's roof; dripping, oozing and running down the wall of the house onto the garbage bag it rested on. In my opinion, the sugar entered each child's bloodstream at exactly the same second, and we were pretty much screwed from that moment on.

When the doorbell rang, Max and Bryn ran to see who was there. I opened the door and happily signed for two packages. Must be Christmas gifts from Tanya and the gang in the Maritimes, I thought. Since there were two boxes, it was perfect. Bryn could open one and Max the other. Erin had gone upstairs to tuck Dana in for a nap while all of this commotion took place. I had the kids come into the kitchen to open the gifts. We all wondered what could be inside. How exciting!

I felt the excitement of the children, and loved seeing it all through their eyes. Everything about the Christmas season is thrilling to a child. The boxes were opened and soon the cousins were flinging beautifully coloured paper shavings all over the floor, hunting for the gifts inside. It did strike me as odd for a brief moment that each box was the exact same size. It looked like each one would contain the same item, whatever that may be. And then it dawned on me.

A couple of weeks earlier I had gone online to check out a website Dave had learned about and passed on for my information. The site was called "Titbits" (www.titbits.com) and was created and run by a breast cancer survivor named Beryl Tsang. After being diagnosed with breast cancer and having a breast removed, Beryl had begun looking for breast prostheses. She was unable to find a product that worked for her. Finally, she ended up knitting herself a soft cotton breast, a "Titbit" as she called it, to use when she got dressed up for a party. She loved the comfortable, light feel of the product, and began knitting "Titbits" for all of the women she knew who had undergone mastectomies.

Needless to say, Beryl had found a niche in the market, creating her website to make the "Titbits" available to women around the world. How fun that you could order them in a variety of bright, fashionable colours. You could order them in cotton, silk or cashmere. You could order them with or without nipples. You could even order them with "nipple piercings" if you were feeling saucy!

So I had gone ahead and ordered myself two pairs; one in basic black and one in practical beige. I had not yet had my surgery, but felt like this was a step in the right direction. I was accepting what was to come and had found a way to have a little fun with it. I thought this Beryl woman must have my sense of humour! Online I was informed that it would take up to six weeks for my "Titbits" to arrive by mail, so I had hit the "send" button and forgotten all about it.

Until Max and Bryn were excitedly opening two matching boxes on my kitchen floor that December afternoon! By the time I realized what was inside the boxes, it was too late. The kids were almost at the bottom of the confetti wrap and soon the "Titbits" would be revealed. Quickly I told them that maybe my Christmas Balls had arrived. I had ordered some nice, knitted Christmas balls and perhaps that's what these were. Each child thought on that a moment and then pulled out the surprise. "Yes!" Max cheered. Tante Marcie's Christmas balls were here! Hurray!

It didn't take long for the kids to lose their interest in my festive "balls". Turns out it had been the wrapping that was the most fun part. They moved on to other, more interesting projects, leaving me standing there, on my kitchen floor, looking at the wrapping and confetti all around me. Yes, there I stood with my balls in my hands.

When Erin returned after successfully getting Dana to sleep, the look on her face was priceless! I can't even guess what the look on my own face was at that moment! I explained it all to her and we shared a good laugh. Someday we'd tell the kids about this, but for now it'd be our little secret.

Ah, the Christmas cheer! Looking back, I wouldn't change a single second of our pre-Christmas family times (not even the botched art projects or embarrassing falsie surprise). It gave Erin and me time to spend as sisters and moms, enjoying each other's company and loving each other's kids. I got to see Erin the mom in action, preparing for a Christmas celebration with her son. I had imagined the kind of mom Erin would be someday and there's no question about it: she has raised the bar high.

Chapter 56:
My Final Chemotherapy Treatment

Chemopaloozapalooza

As Christmas day approached, so did my very last Taxol treatment. I was actually excited about it. I couldn't wait to experience it; I'd look around the chemo suite with the eyes of someone saying goodbye. I'd waited nearly six long months for this day.

As luck would have it (and by now you've probably guessed that the luck was not good) a huge blizzard was headed in our direction and scheduled to be at its worst right on chemo day. By noon on the day before chemo the weather was already bad enough that we knew if we didn't head out for Hamilton soon, we wouldn't be able to make it at all. This would mean rescheduling the final chemo treatment, which would in turn affect the surgery date for the mastectomies. It would also mean not finishing chemo before the important milestone of Christmas. This was definitely not an option. After all I had been through already, a mere blizzard was not going to stop me.

So Shelley and I packed our bags and headed to Hamilton a day early. We endured a slow and white-knuckled drive, but knew we had made the right decision. We stayed overnight at the Hamilton Sheraton and enjoyed their "Sweet Sleeper Beds". The next morning we made the quick drive "up the mountain" and arrived at Juravinski with time to spare. Phew.

After the usual trip to the blood lab and Clinic D, we were off to our final visit to the chemo suite. We knew it was the finale and were in good spirits. Our expectations were very high. Plus, we had grown to enjoy my Taxol days, at least on some twisted level, as a full day with no kids, no household chores, no work, no pressure. It was like a spa day for me, only without the pedicure. As a mother of two young children, when else was I going to be led to a bed, covered in warm blankets and handed food, juice and trashy magazines? To hear my chemo nurse say, "Try to rest" was like my fantasy. You mean sleep? In the middle of the day? For at least three hours? Chemo rocks!

When my number was called, I walked into the chemo room and my eyes automatically scanned the room for Sandy. There she was, saving my bed! I hopped in and we chatted, like friends at a real spa. "So, are you getting a massage, too, or just the Taxol today?"

On Sandra's first day of chemotherapy, the day we met, she had experienced an immediate allergic reaction to her Taxol. As soon as it hit her system, I saw her chest start to turn red and panic in her eyes. The nurses were there immediately, stopping the flow of the Taxol and getting the situation under control.

I can still hear Sandy as she said to the nurse desperately, "Don't stop the Taxol. I *need* this treatment". It broke my heart and scared the hell out of me at the same time. This served as a reminder to me that, as relaxing as my Taxol days were, we were not at a spa. We were there to save our lives. As if your first day of chemotherapy isn't traumatic enough without nearly dying from the drug! As it turned out, she needed to be given far more

Benadryl first and then the Taxol could be started again. Crisis averted. Thank God.

I was too excited to sleep on my last chemo day. I wanted to stay awake, to talk to the nurses, to eat the complimentary cookies and drink the complimentary juice. I wanted to accept the regular offers of warmed up blankets. I wanted to read about Brangelina and Tomkat and whoever else was getting married, having babies and getting divorced in Hollywood. I wanted to look at my arm and really see the chemotherapy going through the tube and into my veins. This was chemotherapy. This was huge. I hoped it was the last time in my life that I would ever have this particular view, from my chemo bed. I wanted to say goodbye.

Shelley and I visited, while Sandra napped from the mega-dose of Benadryl they'd given her earlier. I happened to look up and lo and behold, from around the corner came my Pink Ladies! With balloons! And cake! And gifts! Only my girls would know how special and momentous this day was for me. Each had gone through it in her own life. They *knew*.

I opened the box to peek in at the cake. It was beautifully decorated with a pink ribbon and "Congratulations Ginger" on it. I was moved to tears. I should not have been surprised about the cake, the balloons, and the beautiful gifts. My Pink Ladies were there for me. It was hard to believe we had not known each other for years. Six months of chemotherapy does feel like years, sometimes, so I guess in a way we *had* known each other forever.

On my last day at the chemo suite, my good friend Monica met me there. She had fed her then very young baby, Claudia, and headed for Hamilton. She had wanted to join me on a chemo day ever since I started, but it worked out perfectly that she was able to share this day, of all days, with me.

Monica totally took one for the team that day. Imagine walking in to a very frightening environment, unsure of what to expect. Knowing that no matter how hard you tried to be calm and casual, you would be sitting next to a young woman, a friend, while she had chemotherapy drugs injected into her arm. Not an average day in the life of a thirty-something. After a fun, heartfelt visit, Monica headed home to feed Claudia yet again. Man, babies are so needy. As I watched her walk away, it really hit me how huge it was that she had come. It had been hard for me on my first day there, but already that seemed so long ago.

Monica was experiencing the Juravinski Cancer Centre for the very first time just as I was experiencing it (hopefully) for the last. I wonder if she found it odd how relaxed and comfortable I was there? Believe me - it took a long time to get that way. In any case, Monica's visit is just one of the positive, beautiful things I will never forget about my Chemopaloozapalooza experience. Friends who chemo together stay together.

As my Taxol was coming to an end, and my minutes there were numbered (in a good way), an odd feeling crept over me. Slowly at first so that I didn't completely recognize it. Nope, not nausea. Nope, not gas. Worse. Fear. Suddenly, the thought of walking out of that room, out of that suite, out of that building made me literally shake. I had spent so much time dreaming and fantasizing about this amazing day that I had never ever stopped to imagine what would happen next.

Next? So, I'd drive home. Play with the girls. Make dinner (or, more realistically at that time, eat the dinner that Jeff had either prepared or defrosted for us). Then? Then? I was stuck. How could I walk out of there and just go on with my life, pretending I was back to normal? How could active treatment of my cancer just stop? How would I keep my cancer from returning without chemotherapy? As hard as chemotherapy had been on me, my family and my close friends, it suddenly seemed a much better option than the dreaded *nothing*.

In the end, my Pink Ladies hugged me and bid me a fond farewell. We would keep in touch and "do lunch" from time to time. I knew they meant it. My nurse wished me well. I hugged Sandra in the next bed and we exchanged contact information so that we, too, could keep in touch. She had a couple more Chemopaloozas to go. It was hard for me to picture her getting chemo for one. It had kind of been "our thing". Is that pathetic of me to admit? I know, I know - It's not like we were breaking up.

The drive home was bittersweet. It was huge to be done. A relief. A letdown. Anticlimactic in some ways. Terrifying in many ways. Exhilarating at the same time. Isn't it amazing how many emotions the human brain, even the human brain all hopped up on chemo, can experience at once? It boggles the already tampered-with mind. Big time.

I was brought back safely into reality when I listened to my phone messages. Of course there were messages, what with me never answering my phone. Again, going back to the idea of friends you feel you've always known, I heard Julie's voice and I relaxed. Immediately. Great how some people can have that effect on you.

Julie was asking if I wanted her to deliver my chemo goodies to my house or my sister's house. We had begun calling Shelley's house "The Roehamptons", like a fancy B&B. All of my friends wanted a chance to stay there and relax for a few days, the way I did every chemo weekend. Maybe chemo was an extreme way to get some time off? It worked for me, but I wouldn't necessarily recommend it as the way to go.

Anyway, Julie had baked me fresh banana bread and hand-made a mega fruit salad that was so good even Jeff would eat it. For a while there, I actually thought his scurvy would go away with all the fruit he was eating. No Jeff, barley and hops are not fruit.

Not just once, but on seven of my eight chemo days, Julie knocked on my door with treats in hand. She still apologizes for that one time she wasn't able to feed me. She had just had her beautiful, premature, little angel, Evelyn. That little girl came so close to dying when she was born that we all truly feared losing her. Thankfully, she was a strong wee thing and fought her way back to health with the same strength (and strong will) as her mom.

While Evelyn looked angelic and clearly was a gift from God, she screamed like the devil for the first several weeks (months?) of her life. I could relate to that, as Jeff and I had suspected after Bryn, and then confirmed after Dana, that we did, in fact, make angry, angry babies. Colic was like beer at our house. We wouldn't have known what to do without it.

So when Julie apologized for not showing up that day with a colicky baby in one arm, holding her toddler, Oliver's hand (and a fresh banana loaf) after my first chemo, I laughed and assured her that even Superwoman could not have treated me any better than she had! Maybe, though, I should continue to play upon her guilt so she'll keep feeding us. Note to self: the cancer card is for playing. It has to be good for something.

Chapter 57:
Saying Good bye to My Breasts

These boobs were made for walkin'

On the night before my next big surgery, the mastectomies, I remember that my dad and Dot were there. They were on board to babysit while we were away. Shelley was there, my rock as always. Erin was there, God love her, to keep us all sane and to stay by Jeff's side in the waiting room during my surgery. A good friend and colleague, Sarrah, came by with gifts and hugs and chocolate, which were exactly what I needed at that time. Some people just know what to do and do it.

My sister had prepared a crockpot of chili and there was grated cheese and fresh bread. It smelled great. I sat down to eat and was trying really hard to act natural and pretend it was a regular night. We all were. It was like watching a movie, as if I were not really there. I heard the conversations going on around me but could not focus for the life of me. Perhaps chili was a bad idea. I slid my bowl away from me and left the table at last.

In the end, Jeff and I decided it would be better if we went and slept over at Shelley's that night. Erin agreed that it was a good plan. The girls would be well looked after by Nana and Papa and we needed, *I* needed, to try to get a good night's sleep. Yah - that was gonna happen.

We headed for "The Roehamptons" and were relieved to be out of the house. We visited for a while before I decided it was time to say my last goodbyes to my breasts. I left Jeff, Erin and Shelley in the living room and quietly made my way up the stairs to the bathroom. I leaned over, ran the water (hot!) and chose bubble bath that smelled like candy. It was called "Bliss". That would have to do, since I couldn't find one called "Drunken Stupour" or "Comatose".

While I waited for it to fill up, I sat on the edge of the tub and thought back to earlier that day. Reverend Sue had come to our house to talk to Jeff and me. She offered her support, love and prayers. She spoke openly and kindly about my upcoming surgery, offering suggestions for how to cope with what was to come. She had known other women, other families, who had been faced with the same difficult decision to remove a breast or breasts.

One idea that she mentioned really stayed with me. It was the one in which a woman would say goodbye to her breast(s) before a mastectomy. Sue spoke of the importance of a ritual, a way to mark this important event, and to really allow myself to say a proper farewell. My breasts, she said, had been an important part of my body, my self-image, my sexuality. A part of my identity. My femininity. The breasts play such a role in a woman's life.

Everything she said rang true, and I was secretly relieved to hear her speak of those things. In my mind, before Sue's visit, I had often wondered how I would let my breasts go. How could I just walk into the hospital with two breasts and walk out with none? I felt strongly that I needed to pay my respects. I just didn't know if that was a strange way to feel. Was my need to ritualize this event a sign that I was not coping in a healthy way? Hearing Sue's words, I was at peace with my feelings, my need to spend some time alone with my breasts.

And so I peeled off my clothes, when the tub was full. It's interesting that I recall paying special attention to the feeling of removing my bra. It was the last time I'd remove a bra from my body. I believe I held that bra in my hands for a moment. What would I do with all of my bras after this surgery? Maybe my friend Ceri, an artist, could use them in her creative work? Just imagine the look on her face if I drove up with a box full of bras.

The water was hot on my skin and I smelled the "Bliss" all around me. Or was that my skin burning? In any case, I lay there very still and closed my eyes. I would be fine. I would be fine. I would be fine. Eventually, I found the courage to push the bubbles aside, revealing two breasts that, for the moment, still belonged to me.

I stared at them the way a person would stare at a newborn baby for the first time. I really *saw* them and was brought to tears. I couldn't picture my body without them. Sometimes I think that we become so comfortable with our healthy, functioning bodies that we stop appreciating them. I know, in my case, at least, I had always taken for granted that my body would be whole and beautiful. Healthy and able.

When the wave of tears and emotion subsided for a moment, I had a vivid memory. It was of a conversation with Jeff that I suddenly remembered having not long before we learned that I was pregnant with Dana. I know that this particular memory came to me at that moment for a reason. It was a part of the ritual. A part of the goodbye. A necessary, albeit painful, part of my learning and admitting to myself that I had not always respected or appreciated my body.

Jeff and I were sitting on our bed talking. Bryn was fast asleep and we were getting ready to hit the hay ourselves. We got to talking about how tired we always were. How draining this stage of our lives was. How old we felt. We talked about how difficult it was to find the time and energy to devote to our marriage, our relationship as husband and wife. By the time Bryn was asleep most nights, we had no energy left for each other. Fluffing my pillow seemed like too much work, much less romance and fireworks.

As we shared our feelings openly that night, I recall asking Jeff if he ever wondered if we would some day look back on this time in our lives, this time of good health and happiness (and great, great fatigue!), and regret not appreciating it all more? Did he ever worry that maybe by not making time for ourselves, for not using our healthy bodies more often for comfort, pleasure and closeness, that we would miss out? What if, I asked him then, some day one of us lost our health, and we no longer had the option to appreciate our bodies like we have now? It was a deep conversation, and we both slept fitfully afterward.

Did I have a sixth sense back then that we were about to embark on a difficult journey? Looking back on it from my bubble bath, the night before I lost my breasts forever, I realized with a chill that the cancer had already been in my body at the time of that conversation months ago.

I bathed and paid close attention to my body, to how it looked and felt. I remembered the excitement of seeing myself in a bikini for the first time at 16 years old. I recalled the look on my poor mother's face as I walked out of the change room and spun around, showing off my curves. She said, awkwardly at best, that it seemed to fit OK, but if we bought it I was only allowed to wear it at home, in our own backyard. That, of course, made me want to buy it even more!

I also remembered bra shopping for the very first time, with Tanya and her mom, Susan. Susan drove us to the store, teasing us in a fun way and calling us "The Parton Sisters". We were, of course, at 11 years old, as far from Dolly Parton as anyone could be, but wanted training bras all the same.

The bath water began to cool off and at last I was ready to say my final farewell. I prayed to God to keep me safe, to get me through the surgery without complication and to help me heal. I prayed for help accepting my new body after surgery for what it was; breastless, true, but also cancer-free. I thanked God for the many years of perfect health. For a beautiful body.

Then, I thanked my breasts for their beauty, for being a part of Marcie Elaine Adams. Marcie Elaine Nolan. I told them I'd miss them every day for the rest of my life. But I had to let them go to save the rest of me. And then I pulled the plug.

Chapter 58:
The Bilateral Mastectomies

Making molehills out of mountains

Don't you hate it when you finally fall into a deep sleep after hours of tossing and turning only to be awakened by the shrill sound of the alarm clock? Why is it always so near morning when sleep finally comes? On the morning of my mastectomies, we had set the alarm for very early, given that my OR time was 9 o'clock and we needed to be at the hospital an hour early. When that alarm sounded, my first thought was that we could just do the surgery another time. No biggie.

Then it dawned on me, as I slowly came out of my foggy, sleep-induced stupour, that today was "the day". I had taken my bath the night before, so only needed to splash water on my face and hair. I brushed my teeth. Took my meds. Went downstairs painfully dry-mouthed but forbidden to take even a tiny sip of water. It was going to be a long day.

Shelley, Jeff, Erin and I moved around the house quietly. There was little to say at that point. I guess we all had the same basic thought, "Let's just get this over with". I definitely awoke that day tired but with a sense of excitement. I had been anticipating this surgery for many weeks and was ready to get in there and do it (well, to let the Breast Lady do it, anyway). I truly felt at peace with my decision to remove both breasts, and knew in my heart that it was the right thing to do. I also felt strongly that, having said goodbye, my breasts were already gone from me.

We drove to the hospital, all of us looking out the windows but none of us noticing the trees or houses as we passed them. At the hospital, we signed in at Ambulatory Care. There was an eerie sense of déjà vu, almost as though I'd been there before. Oh, right, I *had* been there before. It wasn't nearly as terrifying this time around. I knew the routine and had let go and let God.

I was shown to my little waiting cubicle, Jeff holding my hand as we followed the leader, and instructed to change into my gown. Then, we were to wait for the nurse to return. I once again paid close attention to my naked self while I got into my gown. Nope. Don't need them anymore. I wonder if Jeff looked more carefully that time, too. It's a topic we have yet to discuss in great detail. Too fresh.

My visitors took turns keeping me company and we all kept an eye on the clock, praying more than anything else that I'd be taken to the OR right on time. The wait went by surprisingly quickly that time, and the next thing I knew, it was show time. I was parked, just like last time, against the wall outside the OR. Either it was freezing in that hallway, or I wasn't as calm as I wanted to believe.

I should mention that on this surgery day I did have an extra sense of security. I am fortunate that Dr. Choong spends some of his time assisting in surgeries. As soon as I knew I'd be having my breasts removed, I called his receptionist, Cathy, and had her book me an appointment with Dr. C. as soon as possible.

I had been anxious to see Dr. Choong anyway. He always gave me a new, better perspective on the events of my life. I had already discussed my options with him at great length, including the bilateral mastectomies, a choice that he fully supported long before the surgery date was set.

The Bilateral Mastectomies

So, this visit was really to ask him, to beg him if necessary, to assist Dr. MacGillivray with my surgery. I knew that I would be well looked after by The Breast Lady, as always, but prayed with every ounce of my being that Doc Choong would be free to be there, too. Just seeing him would put my mind at ease. Hearing from him on the big day that I would be fine and to hang in there would go a long, long way towards keeping me sane.

I realize that it's a gift to have a family doctor who not only knows what he's doing in terms of medical care, but who has taken the time to get to know me as a person along the way. I can't actually picture how the events following my breast cancer diagnosis would have gone if I had had some other, less caring, doctor looking after me. I guess the medical decisions and procedures would have been much the same with a different physician, but I would have missed out on the genuine concern, wisdom, advice and sense of humour that came as part of the Dr. Choong package. Does it sound as if I'm in love with my family doctor? I swear to you I'm not. Not love, but strong, strong like. You will not be shocked to learn that Dr. Choong immediately agreed to be there by my side, assisting Dr. MacGillivray on January 24th. He called "Jeannie" and set it up. We were good to go.

As I lay shivering in my wheelie bed, outside the OR, with some time to pass, I recall feeling very, very calm. I was where I needed to be. This was absolutely the right thing to do. I was a wise, wise woman to have made this decision. Wise beyond my years. And then I waited some more.

Soon, Dr. Choong paid me a visit, asking how I was doing and reassuring me that it was almost time to get on with it. I was

-209-

right. Seeing his trusted, familiar face did make me feel better. Much better. If they could have rolled me in and knocked me out at that moment, I'd have gone in like a hero. Sadly, time went on and I continued to wait, becoming less and less calm. Feeling less heroic. More nauseous, really.

Just as I was revising my escape plan in my mind, I happened to glance down the hall. There, to my relief and surprise, stood Doctor Fraser. He was smiling that smile that is as much in his eyes as on his mouth. He waved at me and I waved back. He stayed where he was and whisper-hollered that they'd kill him if they caught him there. That's Doc Fraser. He has a bit of the devil in him, which makes him all the more fun.

He became very serious all of a sudden. He looked straight at me and told me I was going to be fine. I could do this. I knew he was right (he's always right, remember?). Seeing him at that moment was exactly what I needed. It built me up again. Made me strong. No more panic. No more terror. Just peace within me. And hunger. I was starving and couldn't wait to wake up so I could eat something.

After a quick visit from Dr. MacGillivray, I was rolled into the OR. Doc Choong was by my side, psyching me up. I saw that someone was at work preparing my drugs. That was good. The details at that point become fuzzy.

I relaxed in a way that I wouldn't have thought possible. Maybe it's because I knew my doctors so well and trusted them completely. Maybe it's because I knew that the narcotics were on their way. In any case, I simply know that I truly put myself in God's hands (*and* Dr. MacGillivray's *and* Dr. Choong's, of course) and it felt right. And then the drugs. They also felt very, very right.

Chapter 59:
Recovering From the Mastectomies

Glad I got that off my chest

Bright lights. Lots of voices. Shivering terribly. Yup, this was the recovery room. I'd know it anywhere. A nurse came to my bedside to see how I was doing. "Very well thanks. And you?" When she was satisfied that I was nicely coming out of the anesthesia she gave the porter the go-ahead to roll me out of there. My family was informed that all was well and told they were welcome to meet us in my new room.

I have no recollection of getting to my room. One moment I was in the recovery room and the next I was settled comfortably (comfortably numb, that is) in a bright, clean, private room. Jeff was by my side. I saw relief on his face. As a wife, I had turned out to be a real "fixer-upper," hadn't I? With what we then believed to be my final makeover behind us, we could both rest a little easier. A lot easier.

Let me tell you about my pain medication. I was given a pain pump. It was a contraption that allowed me to push a button whenever I felt pain. Pushing the button would release a safe amount of morphine into my IV. After the lumpectomy experience, I was thinking I would now make up for the lack of pain relief available to me back then. So all I do is push the red button? Cool.

At least it was cool at first. I don't think I overdid it. I used it only when I felt something. Anything. Push. Push. And I slept a lot. People, mostly nurses, I think, came and went, going about the business of checking my vitals and tending to my needs. Good times.

What a relief to be in my own private room. Any room but the OR would have been a welcome change, but this room all to myself was especially good. You see, I still had to look at myself. I could not rest until I took a peek at Doctor MacGillivray's handiwork. I knew my breasts were gone but could not really fathom that cold, hard fact. Without so much as a second thought, I pulled open my gown and looked down. I don't know if I was expecting to hear a drum roll or what, but what I saw was simply me, only different. Flatter.

It is hard to explain the mix of feelings that accompanied that moment. The unveiling of the new me. I was surprised not to see my breasts where they had always been, even knowing as I had that they were gone. If they hadn't been gone, I'd have been in deep trouble. So would Dr. MacGillivray because it would have meant she had removed the wrong body part. I'd hate to have to start calling her "The Leg Lady".

Unbelievable as this may sound, I very quickly came to like the new look of me. My scars did not frighten me. They did not make me cringe. They were already a part of my body and I embraced them more easily than I would have believed possible. I have to give credit where credit is due. The Breast Lady took her time and did an amazing job. I mean, the scars are so perfectly symmetrical she must have used a ruler.

Actually, she did. Or something like that. Dr. Choong had popped in to see me while I was still in the recovery room. He had jokingly said that Dr. MacGillivray had done a very, very, very thorough job. She had painstakingly measured and re-measured me so that both sides would look alike. As I looked at my chest, I was thankful for her. You didn't have to be a genius to see that she did an outstanding job. Once again, The Breast Lady had performed her magic.

The next one to check out the new me was Jeff. We were both anxious to just get the awkward unveiling over with and move on. He took a look and I watched his face carefully for signs of revulsion. Nope. Relief. He, too, appeared to be oddly comforted by the reality of my new look. We had both built it up in our minds for so long that the true scars were not nearly as bad as what we'd pictured.

I don't know if it was the drugs doing their thing or not, but I was feeling very comfortable with my scars. Maybe even a bit proud of myself for getting through this event without curling up into the fetal position and rocking like a baby. I was a very strong woman and I was acutely aware of it at that time.

When I opened my eyes to see my little Bryn standing at the foot of my bed, I was overcome with emotion. I just wanted to leap up and scoop her into my arms. Given that leaping and scooping were not wise things to do at that point in time, I opted instead to have her carefully sit on my lap.

She looked at me solemnly and asked, "Did you have another baby, mommy?" I told her that no, I had not had another baby. I had the two best girls in the whole world and would not be having any more babies. It dawned on me then that the last time Bryn visited me in the hospital was to meet Dana for the first time. Clearly, she associated me being in the hospital with me having babies.

Next, with her main fear being assuaged by my assurance that I was not about to spring another sibling on her, she came up with her next question. "Did they cut them off, mommy?" I told her that the doctors had done a super job and yes, they had removed "them".

Of course, she wanted to see for herself just what "cutting them off" would look like and I felt in my heart that it would be less traumatic for her to just see me right away as opposed to hiding it from her, leaving it all to her own imagination. I knew personally how the imagination could get carried away if we let it. So, I pulled out my gown enough for her to lean over and look down. "Oh, yeah, they did," she said. And then she told me the funny thing she did with Sarah and Kristy at Dianna's that day. Again, we were done talking about it, at least for the time being.

My family and friends headed home when they were certain that I would be fine. I was not in any pain and was still sleepy most of the time. We hugged, kissed and said our goodnights. We would all see each other in the morning. After a peaceful day of dozing off and trying unsuccessfully to wake up, you can imagine the shock I had when my body and my pump turned on me. Let's just say there was projectile vomit involved and leave it at that. All good things must come to an end. "No, nurse, I was not aware that I had an allergy to morphine. Good to know."

I had been punked by the pump. Out it came. Oral meds it was. To be honest, I was not feeling nearly as poorly as I had anticipated. When the nausea and vomiting subsided sometime in the wee hours of the morning after my surgery, I felt really good. I was relieved to be out of surgery. I was relieved to have had yet another complication-free experience in the OR. I had lived to tell.

Chapter 60:
A Visit from Dr. Fraser

Don't worry. Be happy.

At the end of my first day as a breastless woman, before the pump and the morphine executed their plan to attack me violently, I was lying in my hospital bed feeling really good. I was not in any real pain anywhere, which was nice. It was just past dinnertime and I had enjoyed whatever food it was that had been served to me. Food brought right to my bedside. I must remember to tell Jeff about that. I liked food coming to my bed.

It was past visiting hours but too early to fall asleep. I'm not much of a television fan, so wasn't interested in finding something on the tube. I flipped through my trashy magazines, admiring the breasts of all of the stars. Wow, Hollywood is full of large breasts. I guess I always knew that, but that night I really noticed it in a different way. In an "I'm not like them anymore" sort of way (and of course I was *just* like those supermodels before my surgery, right?). With a little airbrushing, I was sure I'd be just fine.

I was getting used to nurses coming and going, so was taken aback when I glanced up and saw Doc Fraser. In he came. He sat in a chair and put his feet up on my bed, ready for a heart to heart.

Doc asked me how I was feeling. I said not bad, what with the drugs and all. Of course he didn't mean to ask how I was feeling, but how I was *feeling*. You know there's a difference, right? It's in the tone of voice. With the "How are you *feeling*?"

question there's often a slight head nod, a gesture that shows the person is digging for a deeper response than the usual surface "Good. You?"

Those who know me well know I'm generally better with the "Good. You?" types of replies, especially when I'm really not *feeling* well at all. I knew what Dr. Fraser was asking and was glad to have him there to talk to. The truth is, I was feeling a bit too "well". I was worried that my denial ran so deep that I just felt like the old me. The "whole" me.

We talked for a long time, just the two of us. We talked about my options regarding breast reconstruction. He knew of someone really great who could do that eventually, after I had taken much time to heal. I told him I thought I'd be fine and that the idea of not having breasts didn't really bother me all that much. It was weird but not the worst thing that could have happened. I was alive and well, had happy, healthy kids and a great husband. I was going to focus on all the good in my life. I know he knew it hadn't all hit me yet. He allowed me my denial for the time being.

Doc F. also asked me about my plans to return to work. He wondered what I was considering in terms of when I'd go back, how many hours I'd work, and what I'd go back to. I honestly answered that I was too tired, sore, traumatized really, to even consider going back to teaching (or anything) in September. I just knew that that was not physically or mentally an option. Not happening. He agreed with me wholeheartedly and encouraged me to take the time to heal, to work through all that had happened to me, to rest, and most of all to take the maternity leave that I had been robbed of. I needed to spend good, long, quality time with both girls. Build up our relationships, deepen our connections. I had not been the energized, active, upbeat mom I used to be, although God knows I tried. It was time to really do the things Bryn had missed out on. I had missed out on them, too.

As for Dana, well, it was time to concentrate my energy on bonding with her. In her first year of life, she had been very loved and cared for, but by all manner of family and friends. She was passed around a lot, fed and changed and bathed by a million different faces and hands, and to be honest, I wanted to be her favourite. I adored her so much, and knew I needed time to show her.

It felt good to say those things out loud to Dr. Fraser. Knowing he supported my stay-at-home decision made me feel less guilty about it. It's hard sometimes, at least for me, to allow myself to do what I want and need. To put everyone else's feelings aside and do what's best for me as a person. Finally I was ready to take time to really heal, in all areas of my life.

I felt we were talking person to person, friend to friend, not just doctor to patient that day in my hospital room. We were bonding. Don't worry; it wasn't the beginning of an affair or anything. This was Guelph, not Hollywood after all. I just trusted him enough to be able to really tell him how I felt, and, lucky for me, he cared enough to sit and listen.

Chapter 61:
Leaving the Hospital

Home, James

I only ended up having to stay in the hospital for two nights and three days, a fact that amazes me still. Aren't people in longer than that for a tonsillectomy? When I was ready to leave, I got up, changed from gown to sweats (carefully, but still, isn't that unbelievable for three days post-op?), packed my bags, went to the bathroom, and called Jeff (not from the bathroom) to tell him I was ready to be picked up. I'm not even sure he believed me at that point.

When Jeff arrived, he found me sitting on the bed, anxiously awaiting my release (although it had been fun to laze around for a few days and to sleep as much as I wanted to. Plus, I've already mentioned the whole food in bed thing. That was great!). He grabbed my bags and the beautiful gifts from my closest friends and colleagues. I hopped out of bed. No, maybe not "hopped". But I did get off the high bed by myself and we said goodbye to the nurses. They had been so good to me.

We slowly made our way to the elevator, headed to the parking lot, loaded up the trunk and got in the car. Jeff kept trying to help me, God love him, but the Adams in me was showing and I was not accepting help from anyone. I was fine, dammit.

I still remember the feeling, or lack thereof, when I fastened my seatbelt that first time in the hospital parking lot. I had worried about that for weeks before my surgery. I couldn't imagine a pain even worse than what I had experienced after my lumpectomy. Wearing a seatbelt had literally never stopped hurting (and I mean real, full-blown pain) since the two lumps had been removed. In my mind, having both breasts surgically removed would have to be even worse. Not true. What a lovely surprise. On went the seatbelt, quite comfortably all things considered, and off we went. Home, James. Well, home, Jeff.

Chapter 62:
Convalescing at Shelley's House

Auntie Bug's B&B

As you know, recovering at my house amidst the chaos of Bryn and Dana, family and friends, would not have been an option. I once again imposed on my sister, Shelley, or, as we like to call her, Bug. My dad used to call her that when she was a wee thing and I guess it just stayed with her. My girls call her Auntie Bug and to us, it's perfectly normal.

So, Jeff pulled into Bug's driveway, unloaded my stuff, helped me get all set up in my sick room and stayed a while until I was comfortable. I don't know who was more relieved to be out of the hospital. Actually, yes I do. He was.

When he headed home to the girls, Bug took over. She had prepared my room in advance, and let me tell you, it was the most incredible room you've ever seen. When she bought her house she opted to use the very large master bedroom as a library. An avid reader, she had always dreamt of a reading room of her own and now she had one.

It was beautifully painted, decorated tastefully with eclectic cat-themed art (not the tacky, creepy kind) and had shelves and shelves of books. I've often thought, while looking around at her multitude of soft-covered, hard-covered, old and new printed tales, how sad it is that her taste in books sucks.

Okay, maybe that's a bit harsh. I kid her about that, but really it's an innocent case of us having completely different tastes in reading material. For Bug, think epics and aliens, sometimes even in the same book. For me, think "What would Oprah pick right now?" It's not that I don't have a mind of my own, but Oprah has yet to recommend a book I didn't love, or at least appreciate on some level or another.

So, I lay in my sick bed, surrounded by hundreds of books I'd never pick up off the shelves. Still, the room felt warm, safe and I noticed a distinct lack of "it". Ah, sweet bleachless air.

I figure that the huge electric fireplace at the end of my bed aided me significantly in my recovery. Seriously, just push the red button to feel hot, and the green one to feel cool. Wicked.

Early in the initial recovery process I quickly came to call my sister's house the B&B. It was like a vacation without the outdoorsy activities. She fed me, propped my pillows, sat with me so we could talk about all manner of things and left me to sleep when I needed to close my eyes.

It was inevitable, I suppose, that my friends, upon hearing about my star treatment, would line up for a room at the Inn. No way in hell was I giving up my spot.

Chapter 63:
Recovery Continued

Paging Nurse Tanya

Well, there was *one* person I was willing to share my refuge with. Her flight arrived at the airport and I saw people coming through at Arrivals. It was just like a movie, really. Our eyes met across a crowded room, we smiled, ran to each other and held each other close. Best friends reunited to face adversity together.

OK, that's not exactly how it happened, but I wish it could have been that way. In reality, I was sore and lethargic, anxious and generally uncomfortable in my skin; in other words, I was in no shape to pick Tanya up at the airport.

Instead, Jeff picked her up for me and delivered her to our front door. I had returned home to my family to await Tanya's return. My kids were delighted to see her and vied for her attention. Jeff had been taking care of the kids and feeding us all, running the household as best he could on little sleep and under tremendous stress, so was noticeably relieved to see her take over.

As Jeff sat on the couch to watch TV, Tanya literally walked through our door, kicked off her shoes, tidied up our family room, fed Dana a bottle and chatted with me while she moved comfortably around my house. She is a master at creating order out of chaos. That woman can clean.

I admit that Jeff, after all he had been through, absolutely deserved, and had earned, a rest. No question there. However, unfortunately for him at that time, I was just learning to heed everyone's advice and take care of *me*. To put me first. Remember how hard that is for me to do? It turns out it's even harder when I see my best friend caring for my kids and doing housework. Again, Jeff was wiped out and desperately needed help. It's just that he would have to call one of his own peeps to help him on this one.

I selfishly decided very early on that this time, I needed Tanya all to myself. I needed time to talk to her, to vent, to laugh and to cry. I couldn't really be myself if we were constantly at my house, where the kids needed us, were watching us, hearing us and hey, let's be real, bugging us.

It was not help with the kids and the chores I really needed at that time, but a safe person to just be with me. To help fill up the space around me. To make the days more enjoyable and nights bearable. The dark of night had, as in the early days after my diagnosis, brought with it sheer, crippling terror. My own voice in my head, going around and around, always coming to the same conclusion: I could not die and leave my kids motherless. And the tears. Rivers of quiet tears.

I believe it was Tanya's second day with us. I was able to move slowly and we took full advantage of my mobility. We shopped, ate out and, of course, had gone to Tim Hortons several times already. I had to move much more slowly and gingerly than normal, and I took more breaks than I used to, but it was so good to be out in the world again.

At one point late that afternoon, I confided to Tanya guiltily how hard it was for me to be at home while recovering. It was difficult to watch others with my kids, caring for them the way I wanted to. It was uncomfortable to just sit back and watch Tanya cleaning my house (although I'd highly recommend her if your kitchen needs a complete makeover). I felt so relaxed away from it all, where I could deal with me. At my house, I was physically and mentally incapable of putting my own needs ahead of my daughters'.

At my house, the mom in me seemed always to take over, making sitting still impossible. Tanya already knew this, of course, before I said a word. That conversation allowed her to admit that she saw a noticeable difference in me the moment I walked through the door of my house. Going in I was a wreck, going out I breathed more deeply. It was time to let go of the guilt of getting sick, of being sick, and to face it.

We opted to face it at Auntie Bug's B&B. A beautiful place with lots of space and the price was right. Tanya graciously took one of the other guest rooms and left me to enjoy the fireplace. It was a sacrifice I appreciated, especially knowing she could have totally taken me in an arm wrestle if she'd wanted to.

As soon as we each put our travel bags in our rooms, we met in the upstairs hallway, looked at each other and laughed. We were free to focus on ourselves. Since Tanya's daughter, Megan, had been born six years earlier, we had never really had a child-free visit. From that point on, we were mommies first, best friends a close second. Or at least that's what we've always told our kids. Joking, joking.

I will never forget that time we got to spend together. We talked about so many things. I shared my deepest thoughts and fears, as did Tanya. We put it all out there. After more than 20 years as close friends and confidantes, you can imagine that there was very little we had to tell each other that came as a surprise.

Yet, after spending more than half our lives together, we found ourselves in uncharted territory. We had discussed our belief in God many times, debating the issues, agreeing and sometimes simply agreeing to disagree. I have always loved our freedom to share our beliefs openly. I respect Tanya so much for her integrity and ability to stand up strongly for what she believes without forcing her views on others. I have never hesitated to tell her about my religious thoughts, awakenings, struggles or doubts.

To take those earlier conversations about faith, heaven, prayer and God to the next level, to that place where it was suddenly very real and perhaps slightly too close to home for us both, was at first unnerving. We delicately wove our way from concepts and ideas to more tangible issues.

I told her I was afraid to die. I believed strongly in God and heaven, so that was not a part of my concern. It was the *act* of dying that worried me. The pain and suffering. The breaking down and failing of my once healthy body. The moment of cross-over from living to dead. Would it be like falling asleep? Would there be a light to guide me or was that only in the movies? Would my mom be the very first angel I'd see? I said that I hoped so. I still hope so.

It was during that very emotional discussion, between tears, nose-blowing and hugs, that Tanya shared with me a dream she had had not long after my cancer diagnosis. She explained that it may very well have been a simple dream, but everything in her demeanor and direct, unmoving eye contact told me she felt it was much more than that.

My mom had come to Tanya in her sleep with a message of hope. She knew that Tanya would soon be visiting me, helping me through my surgeries and chemotherapy. She also knew, as every mom does, how I felt deep inside. I had spoken to her quietly from my bed many a long, dark night. I had confessed to her my fear of dying. My terror of leaving my home on earth. My desperate need to raise my children and share with Jeff the joy of parenthood. In Tanya's dream, my mom looked into my best friend's eyes and said that she was very excited to see me again, but not yet. It was not my time to go but she would wait for me until it was. Many moons from now.

I don't know about you, but who in their right mind would not take comfort in those words? Dream or no dream, and I'll leave you to your own thoughts on that one, my heart filled up and for me, it was real. I chose to believe that it was a message to me, through the one person in the world my mom knew to go to, from Nancy. Mom. I hold it close still, bringing out that memory, playing the scene out in my mind, whenever I am afraid. My mom always did know how to make it all better. As it turns out, she still does.

Chapter 64:
The Healing Properties of Good Food

Crapfest

After a few late nights of tears, laughter and bonding, Tanya, Shelley and I were ready to loosen up and have some fun. Lucky for us, Shelley had arranged a Crapfest in Tanya's honour.

The concept of "Crapfest" may be new to many of you, which is a crying shame. As far as I'm concerned, all women should have or attend regular Crapfests as part of their sanity-saving, self-loving regimens.

As the title would suggest, it is a festival of crap. Let me assure you that no large communal bathrooms are involved, although it's not a bad idea for the end of the night. Anyway, all of your best, favourite, supportive friends are invited to your home. Every member must arrive in sweats, or another form of elastic waistband pants if her sweats are in the wash. No makeup. No big hair (unless it's a bed head).

The cover charge is simply a bag, bowl or Tupperware container full of something chocolaty, cheesy, or both. No fruits or vegetables are allowed, unless, of course, they are to be used solely for the purpose of dipping into something chocolaty or cheesy.

So, the rules are simple. If you follow them, you will be welcomed with open, flabby arms. If you break them, you will be shunned. Pointing and laughing will be involved. You make the call.

Putting the physical details aside for a moment, I feel it is worth telling you about the mental benefits of a full-on Crapfest.

Do you have any idea how freeing it is to be amidst a roomful of beautiful, loving women of all shapes and sizes? To sit with them, elastic waistband pants stretched to their limit, and feel accepted? Appreciated? Bloated? Okay, the last one is not so much a benefit, but I'd be lying if I left that reality out of my story.

I wish I could take credit for masterminding the first-ever Crapfest, but I cannot. My sister and a group of her closest friends and colleagues had decided one day around the work lunch table that they could all use a night out. Not to some noisy bar. Not to a movie that would force them all to sit in silence for two hours, but to *where?*

Soon the first Crapfest was born. The lovechild of a bunch of women in search of self and peer-acceptance, a safe place to be themselves in a women-only environment. A place to freely talk about their husbands and partners. And a table full of 100 percent pure junk food.

A home was chosen. A date and time followed. The details began to sort themselves out. The rules were easily agreed upon. No guys. Lots of crap. They would only ingest treats for the entire night. Wine to wash it all down with would be made available by the host.

Lucky for me, I had connections to these women. Through my close relationship with Bug, I had inched my way into her "inner circle" of friends. It was both an honour and a laugh-riot to be invited into their circle of fun.

After the thrill of attending my first Crapfest, I went on to attend many more. I loved telling all of my own friends juicy tales from the crap table. I admit that certain stories told at the Crapfest must stay at the Crapfest (an unwritten but golden rule), but I leaked enough information to gain the curiosity and interest of women everywhere.

When the day of the special guest Crapfest arrived, Shelley went to work and Tanya and I were giddy with the plans for that evening's festivities. We planned our food offerings and chilled the drinks. We straightened up the already spotless house and waited impatiently.

It was then that I gained a whole new respect for Tanya. I've told you about her melty cream cheese-filled puff pastry, right? That was child's play. To watch her make her special Skor Bar Squares is nothing short of magical. How could something so easy be so good? And by good I mean bad. Nope - no veggies in that dish.

The doorbell rang several times and we knew the games were about to begin. In walked Shell, followed by Jill, Jane, Ceri, and Carol. Introductions to Tanya were made and we all got down to the business of warming cheeses and pouring chocolate covered sugar in all its forms into large bowls.

As we sat around the coffee table waiting for our Chinese food to arrive (yes, I admit it. We also ordered enough Chinese food to feed an army that night), the laughter of women filled the air. We were all friends. All equals. All drunk (except for the designated drivers, of course).

The conversation naturally made its way to my health. The Crapfesters had not yet seen me in my breast-free form. They all said they were happy to see me looking so well (and eating so well. Nope - no loss of appetite happening that night). I had chosen not to wear my knitted Christmas balls as breast stand-ins, rather opted for the "au naturel" look. I had been anxious to get the first glances out of the way so that the focus could get off of me and onto someone else.

As it turns out, the focus was never really on me for very long. It was on the heaps of food all around us. What had I been thinking? As if my breasts, or lack thereof, would be noticed much in a roomful of hungry women in large pants. I enjoyed the opportunity to just be myself, whoever I had become over the events of the last months. Among my Crapfest friends, I continued to be simply Mar, not Cancer Mar. If any one of them was uncomfortable in my presence at any point throughout my journey with cancer, she did not show it, bless her heart.

Needless to say, the Crapfest was a huge success. Tanya was voted in as an honourary member instantly. A gal who could eat like the rest of us without shame and who was as much against thong underwear as we were was a welcomed addition to the club.

At the end of the night, a few things were unmistakably clear: I had an amazingly supportive sister, I had amazingly supportive friends, and you have to wear elastic waistband sweatpants to a Crapfest for a reason. Enough said.

Chapter 65:
Shopping for Breast Prostheses

Boobs R Us

As tempting as it was for Tanya and me to just hole up in the B&B forever, we did manage to venture out from time to time. We spent lots of time with my girls, visited with Jeff now and then (although I suspect he preferred us nattering away incessantly over at the B&B) and even saw the light of day a time or two.

My mind had been turning over all of the possible uses for Tanya. I had to make sure that I got anything creepy or medical out of the way while she was still around to go with me. Once she got back on that plane to Halifax, I was on my own again.

At one point, probably while sipping an extra large half and half at a Tim's somewhere, Tanya asked me delicately what my boob plan was. I explained that on one level I was just happy to have my surgery over with and to be healing from it. On another level, I knew that I would need to check out the world of the dreaded "faker".

The breast prosthesis. What a gross word. Thinking about it hardly makes you want to run out and buy a bikini, does it? I had asked about it once while picking up a prescription at a pharmacy downtown. Attached to the pharmacy is a medical supply centre staffed by a woman who is trained to professionally fit women for breast prostheses. I remember telling her that I was curious about "the whole breast prosthesis thing". Very mature, aren't I? She asked whom I knew that would be needing them, and I (again, very maturely) drew her attention to my then still regular-looking breasts and said "these have got to go".

She explained kindly that she had a whole "boob room" in the back (maybe not her exact words) that I could have a look at. Generally it was recommended that a woman wait for a good two months post-mastectomy to be fitted for her prostheses, to allow the body to fully heal, for any swelling to go away and for the chest area to take on its new form (or lack thereof).

She happened to be free at that time and invited me to take a quick peek, even though I still had not even had my surgery. I calmly followed her through a little hallway and into "the room". I smiled, listened to her as she began to tell me my various options (size, texture, colour, nipple, blah, blah, blah). What a kind woman. Too bad the whole time she was talking the voices in my head were busy humming an a cappella version of The Lion Sleeps Tonight. Don't ask me why it was that song they chose, but it was very effective at blocking out the scary stuff.

I told her I didn't need to see any of "them" just yet. I'd do a full tour closer to the time when I'd be needing "them". I don't remember exactly what happened next, but believe I may have actually run from the boob room, definitely before she had a chance to open one of the boxes, into the safety of the main reception area. I vaguely recall thanking her, telling her I'd call her to make an appointment for a proper fitting once I had healed for two months post-surgery and she gave me her card. Thank you. Have a great day. I have to go and poke out my eyes and ears now. Buh-bye.

So you can imagine that, when Tanya offered to go check out the prosthesis place with me, to *really* check it out (no music in my head this time), I was scared but could not turn down the chance to have her by my side and do what needed to be done (again, only properly this time).

We headed downtown. I have no idea what we talked about on the way, but I know it wasn't breasts. She has a good gift for knowing when to allow a bit of denial to flow between us. That was one of those times, for sure. We pulled into a parking space, walked casually up the street to the medical supply store. I pointed and said, "This is it". She said, "Cool. Let's do it". In we went. I re-introduced myself to the Prosthesis Lady and off we walked down the dark hallway.

In a movie, that would have been the part where you'd have seen a glowing neon light coming from underneath the closed boob room door. In our case, it was much less dramatic. The lady opened the door, turned on the light and began a much more detailed version of our earlier lesson. In the jungle, the mighty jungle, the lion sleeps to ... focus, Marcie. Focus.

I believe I mentioned earlier how Tanya and I have a nasty habit of laughing inappropriately in uncomfortable situations. Is boob shopping with your best friend considered an uncomfortable situation? You betcha. Now not only was I trying desperately to stifle the music in my head, but also to avoid eye contact with Tanya at all costs. One glance and we were both going down.

We were handling ourselves very maturely under the circumstances until it was time to take a look. And feel. The first box was opened and the lady pulled out a prosthetic breast and handed it to me. This was going to be even harder than I'd imagined. On so many levels.

I held the breast form gently at first, barely able to look at it and tried to hand it back. No luck. Gee, maybe the Prosthesis Lady had done this before? She was clearly prepared for me to feel uncomfortable, at least at first, with the reality I was facing and feeling. Literally.

She explained what I was looking at and feeling. What it was made of. What size that particular one was (the size Jeff would beg me to order, but about three times larger than what I knew I'd be getting). I wanted to have breasts again, not audition for a role on Baywatch. She showed me how that one actually stuck to the palm of my hand when I turned my hand over. That is a popular feature so that when a woman puts it on (on her chest, not her hand, just to clarify) it doesn't feel as though it is going to slide around or fall off.

Then she did the inevitable and yet unthinkable. She asked me to hand it to Tanya so she could feel it. Watching my best friend feel me up from across the room also fell into the category of terribly awkward, and terribly funny. You have likely grown to feel you have known Tanya for as long as I have, so it shouldn't be a shock to hear that she didn't miss a beat before making some off-the-wall comment about my nice jugs. Or jug, anyway.

We laughed and laughed, and thankfully our helper that day had a great sense of humour. Once we got it out, we both were much freer and more comfortable to go about the serious task of figuring out what would be best for me. This was not, we both knew, a joke. Funny, yes. A joke, no. I would really need to make a decision at some point and get on with my life as a woman with breast prostheses.

By the end of our appointment, we knew all we needed to know to make an informed decision. My two months of healing were far from over, so the decision could wait a little longer. What could not wait any longer was lunch. Who knew that breast shopping could make a gal so hungry? Comfort eating? Nah. Over lunch we took some time to really talk seriously about my decision, what information we had taken in and what I might end up actually doing. Again, when someone knows you really really well, you can easily go from kidding around to deep and meaningful as required.

That was enough excitement for one day, so we paid the bill, headed home, changed into sweats worthy of a Crapfest, and vegged in front of the TV. At one point, we spoke sadly about how it was almost time for Tanya to go back to the Maritimes. She looked at me and asked, "So, are you going to show me your scars?" Interestingly enough, I had wanted to show them to her. I had felt like I just needed her to know how I looked. I knew she would be OK with it. I just hadn't been sure if it would have seemed bizarre or morbid, or just plain wrong, for me to offer to flash her. As it turned out, Tanya needed to see just as badly as I needed to show her. It's a best friend thing. I lifted up my T-shirt so Tanya could admire the Breast Lady's work and she didn't even show the slightest bit of discomfort. We spoke very little about it, but I am certain that we both felt much better for having shared that extremely personal moment.

Then we just sat on Bug's couch for a while without speaking. A comfortable silence between friends is one of my favourite sounds in the world. I recall thinking to myself that I was so profoundly lucky to have Tanya's love in my life. While I hadn't thought it possible for us to get closer than we had been before that visit, it was evident that our friendship had just been catapulted to the next level. I thank God, again and again, for nurse Tanya. As always, she had managed to "heal" me in all the perfect ways.

Chapter 66:
Getting the Tubes Out

What a draining experience

Once Tanya returned home, I continued to recover a little bit more each day. There were days of great pain. There were days of relatively little pain. It was like a roller coaster, up and down.

Over time, I became more accustomed to the feeling of healing. It became easier to look in the mirror without being shocked at what I saw, at who I had become. I learned to bathe myself in the tub without getting any water on my steri-strips. I could dress myself slowly. I could walk, gingerly at first and then, eventually, with less and less painful reminders of the new me.

I wish I could say that I learned to accept my drainage tubes as a necessary part of the recovery process, but that would be a lie. A big one. I generally used deep denial as my coping mechanism. If I didn't look at them, they weren't there. It's not that hard, really. I closed my eyes every time my sister squeezed out the vile liquid. To Bug, it was a game. I had been told at the hospital that the drains would come out once the amount of liquid decreased significantly. That, they said, could take a few days or weeks. Everyone heals differently.

So, at draining time, Shell would squeeze the tubes, each one into a different measuring cup (not the ones she uses to bake) to see which side was "winning". I can only imagine how desperately each side of my chest wanted the darned tubes out, so they fought a good fight. In the end, it was a very close race.

Once both sides had all but stopped leaking, it was time to return to Ambulatory Care to have them removed. As much as I wanted them out, the thought of them being removed was not as exciting as you might imagine. I knew, from experience, that they would be pulled out. The tube I had had removed after my lumpectomy was a thin little thing, and I had barely felt it leave my body. That knowledge comforted me.

Shelley and I sat outside the hospital room awaiting a nurse's call. At last, it was my turn. I looked at Bug and she wished me luck. I went into the room and was asked to sit on a bed with my legs hanging over the side. I was given the usual gown and asked, of course, to put it on so it opened in the front. With that, I was left alone to disrobe.

When the nurse returned, she had my chart in her hand. By that time, I imagine, it read like something out of a Stephen King novel, all blood and gore and suspense. She looked at me closely and said, "You can't be very old from the look of you". True. I told her my age and she shook her head, looking at me then with that same disheartened expression I had learned to expect each time a new person heard my story.

She explained how she would first disinfect the area, and then remove the tubes, pulling each one out. She warned me that I may feel a pinch but it wouldn't be too bad, and it would happen quickly. I told her not to worry. I had already had one tube removed and it had not been nearly as awful as I had imagined. Oh good, she smiled. Then she pulled.

If I could give you some free advice at this point, it would be to always assume the worst in any situation, at least in any situation in which a tube in your body needs to be removed by hand. I had felt far too relaxed and comfortable with what was about to happen that, when the time came, it was a horrible, ugly, rude awakening indeed.

So, in this case, size did matter. These tubes were much larger than the little one after my lumpectomy. Clearly, there is a difference not only in their size, but in how much skin heals onto the tubes. A bigger tube, it seems, has more area for skin to grab on to. Hence, when the tube is removed, there is more skin to be ripped off the tube as it makes its exit. Gross.

In addition to the shock of the pain involved in this process, I also made the mistake of watching the tube come out of my body. I could see in a mirror the large, fat tube literally sliding under my skin and coming out. I can still see that image in my mind's eye. In retrospect, it was a bad idea to look in the mirror at that moment in time. Note to self: if in doubt, close eyes.

Thankfully, once the tubes were out, I was instantly fine (except for Shelley needing to run around the hospital in search of a cold glass of water for her weak-stomached sister). OK, so I guess I wasn't "instantly" fine. But I was fine. There was no pain, no feeling at all, once the tubes were gone. The relief of not having to drag those around under my shirt all the time was huge. I felt much freer and more mobile.

Yet another item off the creepy to-do list.

Chapter 67:
Shelley's Tattoo

Sisterly love

While I was at The Roehampton's B&B recovering, I didn't realize at first that my sister was, in fact, recovering and in pain herself. The day after I voluntarily checked myself in at Shelley's house, she told me she had something to show me.

I was intrigued. I thought maybe it was some new magazines she had bought for my perusal, or a new DVD, or some relaxation music. She's very thoughtful that way, so it wouldn't have surprised me if she had done any of those things. What she did show me, however, *did* surprise me. Big time.

She leaned in close and pulled up her sweater sleeve, revealing the most incredible thing I've ever seen. Okay, even knowing her as well as I did, I did *not* see that coming.

Shelley explained to me, as I felt tears slowly filling up my eyes, that on the night of my mastectomies, she left the hospital and drove downtown in time to make it to her appointment at Stigmata, a tattoo place that is highly regarded in these parts. As it turns out, Shelley had felt so helpless that she wanted to somehow show me how much she loved me. She wanted to experience physical pain, knowing that I was going through so much of it myself.

There are no words for the particular tattoo that my sister chose. She designed it herself, taking her sketch to Stigmata with her. You see, no one had ever requested this tattoo before, or any quite like it. Around her wrist, there is now a permanent pink bracelet and ribbon: the symbols of hope for a breast cancer cure. On the bracelet are the words Hope, Courage and Love. As if that were not spellbinding enough, the letter M, for Marcie, of course, was tattooed in the center of the ribbon.

I stared at it, dumbfounded, overwhelmed and so full of love that I thought my heart was going to explode. Literally. Her wrist was still very sore, very red and only beginning to peel. It would take a long time to fully heal but I couldn't imagine it looking any more perfect than it did that day. However, once healed, that tattoo became the most beautiful piece of art that I had, and have since, ever laid eyes upon. I'm not biased at all. It really is amazing.

Along with feelings of love and adoration, awe and incredulity, I also admit to experiencing a certain level of fear once the reality of what she had done, the sheer magnitude of her sisterly gesture, sank in. No pressure on me to top that gift if, God forbid, Shelley ever found herself in the hospital for any reason! Clearly a Body Shop gift basket was not going to cut it. So, for many reasons, I am thankful for my sister's generous spirit, creative flair and humungous heart. I am also thankful for her, so far, perfect health (knock on wood).

Chapter 68:
Dad's Tattoo

If I'm dreaming, don't wake me up!

I'm guessing you've already figured out by now that I totally have the best sister on earth and possibly the heavens. Now get this; sometime after my sister surprised me with her tattoo, my dad arrived with a surprise of his own.

You have to have a little background information on Don Adams to fully grasp this surprise. I, having been a teenager who knew everything about everything, had made it particularly difficult for him to teach me anything while I was growing up. However, certain lessons were covered regularly enough to sink into my adolescent skull: all boys were bad, but, as far as the evil boy hierarchy went, the lowest of the low were boys with long hair, tattoos or earrings. Dropouts were right up there, too. Needless to say, for a few years at least, my dream boy was the guy with all of the above. If he had multiple piercings, then all the better. Not that I was attracted to anyone fitting the above description, but I dated a few just for the fireworks it created at home.

Anyway, the good news is that dad and I have both come a long way since those tumultuous years, and we are each able to look back on our ups and downs and laugh. Especially him. If you knew my two strong daughters, you'd understand why my dad is presently in "Papa's glory". He gets to play with and spoil my girls anytime he chooses and to leave them anytime he chooses. He can sit back and laugh at their misadventures, too.

All the while, he knows in the back of his head that I, too, will be that strict, uncool, frustrated and often bewildered parent I once judged him to be. That sucks for me, but is hilarious and very satisfying for him.

Now, you can imagine my surprise and shock when dad unveiled his own tattoo. On the back of his right shoulder he proudly displays (weather permitting, of course) the same pink ribbon tattoo with my first initial, M, on it that Shelley has (minus the bracelet). I can truly say that I never, not even in my wildest dreams, thought I'd live to see my dad with a tattoo! The only thing more shocking than that would have been for him to have revealed that he had grown his hair long, all the way down his back! Once again, I was nearly brought to my knees with the loving (and permanent) nature of his surprise. Now that took guts! How in the world did I manage to pick both the best sister *and* the best father a girl could ask for? Clearly my luck isn't always bad.

Mine is not to question why. I will simply remember to remain thankful for and appreciative of the unlimited supply of love and support of my family. How I came to deserve them, I may never know.

Chapter 69:
Depression and Cancer

"If the darkness knocks on your door"

I feel it would be lying by omission if I chose not to spend some time talking about the very real, very difficult issue of depression and cancer. Whether you have any past history of depression or not, a cancer diagnosis, the side effects of chemotherapy, and healing and adjusting to physical scars is enough to bring a person down. Way down.

I'm not talking about the obvious fact that a cancer diagnosis and all it entails sucks. It is sad. It is maddening. It is unfair. It is terrifying. But it is much more than that for many people. I'm not a doctor nor do I pretend to be, so my experiences with depression over the past year are just that, my own personal experiences. I can't speak for anyone else, but I'd like to tell you what I know about *my* depression.

It is not always easy to figure out that you are clinically depressed when you are dealing with something as devastating as breast cancer. You get used to feeling scared, tired, angry, and all manner of negative emotions, on a regular basis. It makes sense that a person would break down in the early days following a life-threatening diagnosis. Add in a colicky newborn, and an active, spirited toddler, and the term "rock bottom" takes on a whole new meaning.

For me, it was not until some time had gone by that I began to see a pattern to my moods. I noticed that many of my crying spells did not occur at a "low time". I was often just watching

TV, folding some laundry and enjoying the quiet sound of Dana napping upstairs. Feeling pretty well, all things considered.

And then the tears would come. Sometimes I cried for a few minutes and other times for two hours steadily. Regularly I would find myself crying off and on all day and into the night. No rhyme or reason. I knew something was not right when I found myself crying all the way through an hour of the Ellen Show. Not tears of hysterical laughter, which would be perfectly normal. Tears of uncontrollable sadness.

Another telltale sign that took some time for me to recognize as a symptom of depression was a bout of insomnia that lasted literally for months. As tired as I was both physically and mentally at the end of each difficult day, particularly during my six months of chemotherapy treatments while Dana was still a colicky newborn, my head would hit the pillow and I would wait for sleep to come. It never did.

I remember fantasizing about sleep sometimes during the daytime. I'd watch the clock, counting down the hours until I could get the girls to bed and hit the hay myself. Time after time I convinced myself that *that* night I really would fall, and stay asleep only to be disappointed once more. I was just so tired. Why couldn't I sleep?

Depression, of course, does not exist in isolation. My ups and downs, tears and tantrums affected my whole family. Poor Jeff was in a houseful of feisty females, from one colicky baby to a headstrong toddler and then finally to a wife he had long since ceased to recognize as the woman he had once known.

Jeff had been home on parental leave for some time since my mastectomies and was planning on remaining home until mid-July. This gave him lots of time at home to spend with his gals. Lucky Jeff. If he at one time had believed that his parental leave would be a six-month holiday, he had been rudely dropkicked into reality. While most men his age may have been fantasizing about Pamela Anderson, I wouldn't be surprised if Jeff was busy fantasizing about a long day at the office. Sweet overtime.

My daughters did not escape unscathed by my depression either. Sadly, they saw my ups and downs, as hard as I tried to shelter them from my emotional roller coaster. I began each day promising myself that I would remain calm and collected, being the kind of mom that I had been raised by. The kind of mom that I thought I was before the whole cancer bomb exploded.

I admit that many days went by with me going through the mommy motions, changing diapers, warming bottles, serving grilled cheese sandwiches for lunch with ketchup on the side, as always. As needed. Yet, in truth, most of the time I did things by rote, but my brain was not there. My heart really wasn't in it, either.

I loved my girls, my husband and my life, at least as it had been, but I dreamed of freezing my family somehow and crawling into bed, pulling up the covers and closing my eyes. For a long time. If I could have put my babies in a bubble to keep them safe from harm, in a way that they'd stay exactly as they were until I could get it together, I would have.

All I wanted was to be left alone. To have no one to care for. No one to cook and clean for. No one to see me suffering. No one to make me feel like a bad wife, a bad mother, a bad person, for having nothing left to give. I really did feel like I was disappearing into a hole so deep no one would ever be able to pull me out. If this was how life after cancer would be, I felt my family would be better off without me. I never considered suicide, but I regularly fantasized about leaving everyone and everything behind and driving far away, to a place where no one knew me. I just wanted to be all alone.

Chapter 70:
Seeking Help for My Depression

The sun'll come out tomorrow

After waiting a long time, hoping desperately that the sadness would cease and the sleep would come naturally, I finally gave in and accepted that I could not deal with my emotional issues alone.

I spoke to Dr. Tozer at one of my appointments and he referred me to the Support Services Department at the Juravinski Cancer Centre. As it turned out, along with first-rate cancer care for the physical realities associated with the disease, Juravinski also offered a variety of free counselling and related services.

Initially, I was contacted by a social worker named Linda. She called me to set up an appointment and we decided that a phone meeting would work best for me at that point, what with the baby and all. Easier for me to talk by phone when Dana took a nap.

When the phone rang on our appointed day at the agreed upon time, I was sitting by the phone. I was so ready to talk about this. Jeff was working from home, so was willing to keep an ear out for Dana should she wake up. I was in the basement at the computer desk, with a notepad and pen. I hoped to take notes, jotting down anything at all that Linda suggested I try to help me feel better.

I knew instantly that Linda was good at what she did. She was very calm, friendly and able to ask just the right questions to help me unload all that had been building up inside me for weeks on end. Many times I broke down mid-sentence, crying as I spoke about my feelings.

I remember that it was especially difficult for me to talk about my daughters. Bryn more than Dana. I felt guilty about Dana not having much of a mom for her first months in this world, but I comforted myself with the thought that she was, thankfully, too young to remember any of this.

Bryn, on the other hand, had been used to quite a different mother than the one I had become. I was afraid I'd never feel well enough to live up to her expectations. It broke my heart literally to the point of tears every single time I looked at her. Every time she spoke. I knew it wasn't healthy for her to see me that way.

I have since spoken to many other moms who have battled cancer too. It seems to be a very common thread among us to have feared disappointing our kids at different stages of the cancer experience, or, worse yet, to die and leave them motherless, with only the most recent memories of us feeling sick, tired and grouchy to remember us by. No mother wants her child to be left with only cancer-related memories when she's gone.

So I let it all come tumbling out, and Linda listened with empathy and insight. After nearly an hour spent this way, she concluded (as she surely did after only five minutes with me on the line) that I would benefit greatly from a meeting, in person, with the cancer centre's psychiatric nurse, Barb. I agreed whole-heartedly. Now that the floodgates had been opened, I knew I needed to keep at this until I found some kind of resolution and peace.

It was not long before I found myself back at Juravinski, but this time in a whole new department. It was on the second floor, like the chemo suite, but in a different area altogether. The Support Services receptionist, a friendly young woman I would get used to seeing, told me to take a seat and she would page Barb to let her know I had arrived.

As soon as Barb walked up to me, I felt relieved. This woman could surely help me get myself together. She, like Linda (and everyone else I'd met in that place) had the perfect way with me. Clearly, she had done this before! It's easy to get so caught up in our own lives that we forget how common our experiences and feelings really are.

We sat together in Barb's little office and I once again began to put my true feelings out there. This time I was even more of an emotional wreck than I had been on the phone with Linda. I hadn't really expected it to be that hard. It was speaking about Bryn, as always, that made me come completely undone.

Barb strongly recommended that I meet with the on-staff psychiatrist after explaining to me that I was very probably dealing with clinical depression, not "just" the usual cancer-related stress. I don't mean to sound as though I'm making light of the usual cancer-related stress. That, too, is very, very bad. In my case, however, there was more.

Since Barb had taken extensive notes at our meeting and typed up a detailed report, the psychiatrist, Dr. Mancini, had lots to go on before I even opened my mouth. I think she probably took one look at me, as I sat in Barb's office with both of them, and knew that it was a textbook case of clinical depression. I was pale, had bags under my eyes (the chemo didn't help with that at all) and just sitting there I could feel my eyes brimming with tears.

I walked out of that office with a prescription for sleeping pills and anti-depressants. I felt better already, just knowing that it wasn't me imagining things. It wasn't me just feeling sorry for myself, either. I try hard not to do that. This was not something entirely in my control, at least in the sense that I knew I couldn't just suck it up and get over it by thinking positively.

Thinking positively would be much easier once I got the new medication into my system. Once my chemicals were balanced. I couldn't wait to fill my prescription and start the process of helping myself get better. It can be very empowering to admit to yourself that you need help, to ask for what you need and to receive it. I recommend everyone try it sometime. As they say, "Ask and you shall receive".

That medication was a huge step in the right direction for me. I had needed help. I slowly began to feel my head coming up out of the sand, and hours, then eventually days and weeks, went by without tears and anxiety attacks. I slept, at least sometimes, and, in a matter of weeks, could feel the benefits of not being physically exhausted and emotionally scrambled.

Due to a long personal history of depression prior to the cancer diagnosis, I know that I will never just stop being depressed. I will treat it and cope with it and tweak things as needed, but I will not wake up without it. Some days, no matter how hard I try to think positively, I am followed by a menacing dark cloud, always threatening my mental well-being and sense of calm.

On those days, I talk myself through all that I have overcome. I remind myself that I have been to hell and back. I also try to be kind to myself, to that part of me that needs a bit of extra cheese to be comforted. A day here and there to just feel sad and anxious is to be expected. I have newfound confidence in the future, in my future and my ability to experience happiness like everyone else. It may take medication, therapy, lots of sleep and, yes, macaroni and cheese, but depression can be kept at bay. It is simply a part of my daily routine. Get up. Brush teeth. Make bed (OK, I don't always make my bed, but I always put it on my "To do" list). Hug kids. Drink coffee. Take meds. Be happy. Drink more coffee. I'm a firm believer that without my antidepressant medication, my daily "To do" list would be much more difficult to manage and less satisfying.

Chapter 71:
The Reach to Recovery Program

Pick up, pick up, pick up

As I neared the end of my cancer treatments, I found myself settling in to a vague routine. Get up. Get the girls ready for their day. Drop them off at the daycare. Drop Jeff off at work. Drive home. Shower (on my better energy days). Put on clean sweats (on my "let's raise the bar a bit" days). Sit and think. Think. Think. Think.

I wasn't ready to go back to my old life, but I wasn't content to simply be the "cancer recovering survivor" that I had become. I wanted to talk to someone else who knew how I felt. It was over as far as the world was concerned. No more chemo dates. No more surgery dates. No more cancer. Done. Move on. So why couldn't I just move on?

I called the Canadian Cancer Society and was put in touch with a woman in charge of a great peer support program. It was called Reach to Recovery, a volunteer program for women recovering from breast cancer surgery. I was asked some information about myself, my diagnosis and some details regarding what kind of support I was looking for. I was told that a match would be found for me based on my own personal story. The goal was to find me a match with a past cancer history as similar to mine as possible.

Three days later, at the most, my phone rang. I let the voicemail click in (I *had* learned a bit from my previous telephone experiences so was still screening calls). When I listened to the message, it was a woman named Donna Kincade. She had been paired with me. She was looking forward to talking to me and getting to know me better. She could help. She understood. She had been there.

I called the number Donna had left for me to contact her. We spoke briefly, just long enough for her to say she'd call me right back. It was a long distance number, and Reach to Recovery would reimburse her the cost of each volunteer phone session. I wouldn't have to pay a cent. Isn't it amazing the support that is out there if you only ask? We set a date and time for Donna to call me again, and we exchanged e-mail addresses.

The first time I spoke to Donna I loved her immediately. Some people you click with and she was one of those people to me. I learned that she had been diagnosed in her early thirties, like me. She had had a mastectomy, like me. She had chosen not to have children, knowing that she had a strong family history of breast cancer, like me. Well, I had had children, but that is where our differences ended.

For a long time, I looked forward to her calls. We had chosen Monday nights at 8 o'clock as "our time". I always had the girls in bed and was able to sit and talk freely. The only problem with our phone friendship was the fact that I was not a phone person. Not a small problem, as it turns out. So, many Monday nights my phone would ring at eight on the dot. I would sit and listen to it ring. I'd let the machine pick up. I'd check the message and hear my friend's patient voice. I'd call her right back, apologizing profusely. The truth was, I always looked forward to her calls all day long. I was glad to know we'd be touching base that evening. However, by the time I got everyone bathed, in bed, tidied up the dinner dishes, got myself into my jammies and sat down, my mind would go blank.

Over the course of many months, Donna and I shared our stories, thoughts and feelings. She was extremely easy to talk to. She was full of positive energy and had a wonderful sense of humour. Part of the Reach to Recovery program included arm-strengthening exercises for women to do at home post-surgery. Very soon after having called to access RTR's services, I received a package in the mail. In it was a booklet explaining the importance of daily exercise as part of a recovery program. It described a variety of simple, quick exercises to do regularly to build up arm strength.

I hated doing the exercises, but Donna always asked me if I had been keeping up with them. I just couldn't lie to her, so I was guilted into taking the program seriously! I must admit that those exercises helped immensely, and also provided Bryn and me with some fun games to play, using a ball that had come with the package. Even Bryn asked me daily if it was time for me to do my exercises yet. She looked forward to it far more than I ever did!

Another thing I immediately loved about Donna was that she was a total cat person. We even had that in common. I loved her stories of the various antics her fabulous felines had partaken in. There was never a dull moment around her home with those fellas around! I told her about my children in the same way that she told me about her cats. We loved them all so much!

From the beginning, Donna was able to comfort me with the knowledge that she had been right where I was and survived. She had more than simply "survived". She had gone on to lead a wonderful, balanced life and had had many wonderful life experiences since her own diagnosis and treatments had ended. And she was showing no signs of slowing down! I should mention that Donna was 52 when we met (by phone). She had been cancer free for more than twenty years! How could I not gain strength and hope from her story?

I still consider Donna to be one of my friends, although we have gone our own ways. I know that there are other women out there who really need her the way I did. It wouldn't be right for me not to share her now that I am getting back on my feet. She is so very good at what she does. It is obvious in talking to her that she is volunteering because she loves to do it.

Donna helped me through a difficult transition time and I am forever grateful. From time to time, we e-mail with updates and well wishes. I am determined that one of these days soon, she and I will set a date, time and place to meet in person. I can't wait to hug her and thank her for coming into my life at just the right time. If I were choosing a supportive friend for myself, I'd pick Donna again.

Chapter 72:
My Heart to Heart with Ceri

Permission to write

At some point along the way, one of my Crapfest friends went from "friend" to "confidante extraordinaire" all in one visit. I met Ceri Lamplugh through my sister. They used to work together and kept in touch after Ceri took a major leap of faith. She had left the comfort and security of her permanent job to make her dream come true.

Ceri is one of the most vibrant, creative, "real" people I have ever met. She is full of life, feels things deeply and loves people. To top it all off, she is the woman to call if you want to have your house made into a home but have no clue how to make that happen. Ceri turns houses into peaceful, gorgeous, comfortable sanctuaries and has a blast doing it.

So, my friend took her love of design and décor and turned it into an amazing home business. She took classes and began building a portfolio of her various decorating projects. It was tough going financially and emotionally for a long time, but hard work and faith in herself have paid off. She is never without work and has a reputation for being "the decorator" to call before making any major (or minor) home decorating decisions.

Ceri, working from home and knowing I was at home, had e-mailed me to invite me to her house for a visit. I'd never invite her to *my* house. She wouldn't be able to sit and talk to me without moving furniture around, painting and organizing my cupboards and closets, and imagining the potential if I'd just have the sense to hire her!

We made a date and I arrived right on time. I always looked forward to getting caught up with Ceri, but on this day in particular I needed to talk to her about something. The two of us cozied up on her couch with our extra large double doubles and she asked how I was doing. Bad idea! That was all she needed to say to get me going on about how I didn't know what I wanted to do with my life. Poor Ceri!

I wasn't entirely sure I wanted to go back to teaching. I didn't know if I should make a change. But if not teaching, then what? All I had ever wanted to be was a teacher. I had never considered other options. I loved teaching, or at least I *had*. Having cancer made me question everything. Would I still love it? Would I be able to do it with as much energy and enthusiasm as I always had? I couldn't figure out where my new place in the world should be. What was I supposed to do? Arghhhhhhhhhhhhhhhhhhh! In my defence, she *had* asked me how I was doing, right?

I told Ceri how much I admired her for having the guts to go for what she wanted. The thought of leaving teaching and trying something unknown terrified me. She asked me, if every option was within my power, what would I want to do? What would make me happy? What if money didn't matter? I'd like to go work on that planet.

Surprisingly, even to me, I did not hesitate to answer her. I would write a book. It was the only thing that deep, deep down I had always wanted to do. I hadn't told many people about that before. Saying it out loud actually changed my life. "Then write a book", Ceri said, as if it was the most simple thing ever.

I shared with Ceri a dream I had, not long after my mom died. It was a dream that was so clear, so vivid and so meaningful that I awoke believing it was more than a dream. It had been a visit from my mom when I needed her, when I hadn't even realized I needed her. To this day, I still believe that it was much more than a dream.

My mother and I were sitting on a big towel on the beach, talking and watching the water. The waves were small and mesmerizing. The details of the dream are faded around the edges now after so many years, but the message is fresh. Mom told me I was going to write a book one day and that it would be great. She was certain of this. I told her I wasn't really a writer and she said, "You are".

For years, I have carried that in my heart, sometimes wondering when my dream, my mom's message to me, would come true. Other times I remember feeling sad, almost as if I had let my mom down by never having lived out that dream. But I never really forgot about that visit. That "dream".

One of the many reasons I never really sat down and took my own inner dream seriously was that I didn't have a story. I didn't have a big idea for a great novel. I was a blank slate. I just needed something to write about that would matter. But nothing came to mind.

"Duh." Okay, maybe not exactly what Ceri said to me, but it may as well have been. "Can you not think of *anything* at all that would make a good story? A story worth sharing with the world?" "Duh" (me talking that time). "Not really." So, dear, sweet, patient Ceri spent her time that day telling me how my cancer experience was an amazing story. It was a story that the world needed to hear and that I needed to write.

She had been receiving my e-mailed updates on how I was doing throughout the process and told me she had laughed (and cried) out loud many times. She loved and shared my sense of humour. It was one of the things that had attracted us to each other in the first place many moons ago. It was my ability to laugh in the face of sheer disaster that struck Ceri as an important message to the world, especially to other women who were facing a breast cancer or other life-threatening diagnosis.

Why not, she suggested, write a book about my breast cancer experience? It was a huge, important story that so many people could relate to or learn from. I had managed to see the humour in all manner of negative situations and that alone could give hope to others who found themselves in a similar situation someday.

Talk about a light-bulb moment! Hmm, she might be on to something. Suddenly, I was a writer. I had a story and I was bursting to tell it. As I talked to Ceri that day, I became more and more excited about my book and it seemed to take on a life of its own from that time on. I knew from the time she pointed it out to me that this *was* my story to tell and I would tell it to the world. My mom had known all along. She had given me permission to write that night when she came to me in my sleep. So had Ceri on the day she asked me what I really wanted to do with my life. And I have not stopped writing since.

A few months later Ceri presented me with a gift. It was a painting she had done of me and my mom sitting side by side on a beach towel looking out at the water. It was entitled "Permission to Marmoir". It was an amazing gift from an amazing and talented friend whose support and understanding inspired me to follow and live out my own dream.

Thanks Ceri!

Chapter 73:
The Results of My Genetic Testing

Time to chop down the family tree

After taking my new antidepressant medication for a few weeks, I started to notice the effects. I was feeling better about my life. I was beginning to feel more energetic, a bit at a time. I had even taken Dana out of the house a few times. A good sign.

At long last, I was also noticing that my body was not in so much pain. The worst of the healing after my mastectomies seemed to be behind me. My right arm was doing pretty well in spite of the removal of my lymph nodes months ago. I was continuing to improve my range of motion on both sides by stretching and reaching my arms up anytime I could. Just grabbing the cereal from a high cupboard made a big difference.

I can't say there was never any surgical pain, but it had become bearable and faded into the background. I was getting back on my feet and feeling human again. Almost normal. And then the phone rang. Again. I wish I could tell you that I had the sense that time to run screaming in the other direction, but I did not. I picked up the receiver and said hello. That was a big mistake. Again. You'd think I would have learned by now.

After two previous cancellations due to the geneticist being ill, I was finally given an appointment date and time to meet with a geneticist at the Juravinski Cancer Centre. To be honest, I had largely forgotten about the whole genetic testing issue. I had given blood so long ago and so much had happened since. The results of this test were the least of my worries.

We were unable to find a babysitter for Dana on my appointment day, so Jeff came along to be on baby duty. Shelley came to sit in on the meeting, having a vested interest in the results. More than ever, the information we were about to receive would affect my sister. We may be best friends, but we are also apples from the same family tree.

The four of us drove back to the cancer centre. We were nervous, but in a strange way. It was as if we already knew the bad news. Yes, I had cancer. Had I been predisposed to get it? Maybe. The end result was the same regardless. For one reason or another, cancer had found me.

No matter how often we said to each other that it really didn't matter what the results were, we all knew that wasn't completely true. Yes, it was a fact that we could not reverse my cancer diagnosis, but we were about to find out if Shelley, Bryn and Dana were at an increased risk as well. I prayed that my blue eyes and sunny disposition (haha) were all that my girls had inherited from my side of the family. Just in case. I also prayed that Shelley took after my dad on this one, since it is my mom's side that is riddled with breast cancer.

I recall entering the Juravinski Cancer Centre and taking an immediate left inside the door. I had only been down that hallway once before, and that was when I went for genetic counselling. It was required before I could decide whether to go ahead with the blood test that might identify a genetic predisposition to cancer.

It wasn't long before my name was called. We walked silently (except for Dana, who was being carried by Jeff and not at all happy about it) to the little room and were told that the geneticist would be in to speak to us shortly. Then we waited.

Why do they bother moving you from the large main waiting area to a little private room if the person you are seeing is nowhere near ready for you? It gives people a false sense of hope that they are next in line. Meanwhile, there might be 12 others ahead of you. This appeared to be the case for us that day.

While Shelley and I sat waiting, listening to each other's hearts racing, Jeff excused himself to take Dana for a walk. As is the case with most infants, it was still really all about Dana in her own mind, so the results of mommy's genetic test were far less important than a bottle of milk and an adventure around the halls of Juravinski. Jeff closed the door behind him, no doubt secretly relieved to be out of there.

At last the Doctor of Genetics came into the room and quietly introduced herself. She sat down, clearly uncomfortable to be in my presence. I'm not sure if she ever ended up making eye contact with us that day. In hindsight, not really a good start to the meeting.

She spoke to us at great length (too great, I'd say) about what it would mean if I had either of the two known genetic mutations, BRCA1 or BRCA 2. Then she explained what it would mean if I did *not* have either of the two known genetic mutations, BRCA 1 and BRCA 2. There were statistics. There were numbers, risk factors, percentages, and survival rates to consider. OK, lady, we get it. Now, what's the word?

Finally, after we assured her that no, we did not have any further questions (other than "Is there anyone else here that could be helping us with this?"), she told us she'd open the envelope and look at my results. Come on! Were we supposed to believe that she had not even looked at my results before entering that little room? *Please.* She *had* to have known.

She proceeded to fumble with an envelope from my file and eventually got the "results" out. She took a quick peek, folded it up again, and put it right back into the envelope. Still no eye contact. Still a bad sign. She told us the sheet she had looked at wasn't the one she needed. It was in a different "format" or something. We had no idea what she was talking about but were too frozen in terror to say a word. We just waited, hearts pounding. Thump thump.

Out came another envelope from my file (God help her if there were eight different forms still to open and close) and she went through the same awkward process of opening it up, taking a look and then closing it up again. This paper did not, however, go back into its envelope. Progress. She glanced at me furtively and pretty much whispered to the ground that I did, in fact, test positive for the BRCA 1 genetic mutation.

Tell me I'm not the only one to ever experience *that* feeling. It was the feeling that even though I had suspected for years that there was a genetic predisposition to cancer in my family, especially breast cancer, hearing the news was actually painful, as if it had been a slap across my face or a punch in my stomach. It was as if the wind had literally been knocked out of me. From the look on Shelley's face, she, too, had been shocked to actually get confirmation of what we had both long suspected. Now the ugly truth was out there: someone had, in fact, peed in the family gene pool. Big time.

Man, I was really wishing I had listened a touch more closely to the geneticist's preamble. Turned out I'd be needing some of that information after all. Once we had listened to her final words (which were, to sum it up in my own words, "Sorry about your crappy luck. Call me if you have any more questions"), we got up, walked out, headed for the car and drove home in silence.

So, it was true. My worst fear (OK one of my many worst fears) had been realized. My apple on the family tree had a huge worm in it. Damn. The next question was, how many other apples on our tree were also wormy?

Chapter 74:
The Decision to Have
Yet Another Surgery

Operation Head on a Stick

One of the details that I had heard the geneticist mention loud and clear was that if I *did* have BRCA 1 or BRCA 2, I would be strongly advised to have a complete hysterectomy as well as salpingo-oopherectomy. In English, that means I would need to have my uterus, ovaries, fallopian tubes and cervix removed. Good times.

Not only did the presence of a BRCA 1 mutation highly predispose me to early-onset (pre-menopausal) breast cancer, but also to greater chances of developing ovarian cancer in my lifetime. As if breast cancer at my age didn't suck enough, let's add a whole new level of suckiness.

It was definitely too late to decide *not* to participate in the genetic testing, and deep down I felt empowered (albeit screwed over) to have this information to work with. The bilateral mastectomies had certainly been a good decision. The next decision was like child's play. I knew without hesitation that I would be opting for the preventative hysterectomy, and asking that anything else in there I wasn't using be removed, too, just to be on the safe side. At this point Shelley and I joked that by the time they were done with me, all that would be left would be a head on a stick.

Initially, I recall speaking to Dr. Choong about this latest turn of events. It was both shocking *and* completely expected.

You don't get that mix of emotions very often. We had already discussed this possibility many months prior to receiving the test results. Upon confirmation of what he and I both suspected, I let Dr. C. know that I had already made my decision and was very comfortable with it. As much as I would miss having the opportunity to see Dr. Fraser regularly, I was *so* done having babies.

The only decision I had to make was whether or not to tell Jeff about this. The plan had been for *him* to be the next one to have a surgery. His vasectomy was all but scheduled, in my mind anyway. If I went ahead with my next surgery, he'd be off the hook. Part of me thought that was a total rip-off. Maybe if I didn't tell him about the hysterectomy right away, I'd be able to get him in for his snip and he'd be none the wiser. Would that be so wrong?

Needless to say, Dr. Choong immediately accepted my decision to go ahead with the surgery as soon as possible and told me he'd refer me to Dr. Fraser for a consultation. I was glad to hear that I had an excuse to get Doc Fraser back on my active team again. I knew after Dana was born that I wouldn't be needing his obstetrical expertise anymore, so in terms of a silver lining, this was it.

While awaiting an appointment with Dr. Fraser, I was off to Hamilton to have a follow-up with my oncologist. Dr. Tozer entered the room and immediately spoke to me about the BRCA 1 development. He said that he highly recommended I have the surgery at Henderson Hospital in Hamilton. It had less to do with what surgeon I would have, and more to do with the handling of my pathology after the surgery. The folks at Henderson had more experience working with genetic mutations such as mine. That was all I needed to hear.

I was referred by Dr. Tozer to a gynecological oncologist (say *that* five times fast). She was highly recommended and I knew I would be in good hands. He set it up and I could expect to hear from her people when they had an appointment date for an initial consultation.

Before I saw Dr. Tozer that day, I remember talking to nurse Judy. We discussed what the BRCA 1 thing meant and what my options were in terms of prevention. I'll never forget what she said to me upon hearing that I had decided to have the full-on surgery as soon as I could get OR time. She smiled, shook her head and asked me if I was always that practical and mature. I wish! The whole cancer thing forces a person to be very responsible whether they want to be or not. Still, Judy had said just what I needed to hear at that time. She's good that way.

I decided to keep my appointment with Doc Fraser to discuss the surgery even though by then I knew my surgery would not be done by him. I wanted to get his thoughts and to learn more about what I would be in for. His office called and I wrote my appointment date on the calendar. Knowing that our meeting was set up made me feel better. He'd tell it to me straight and get me psychologically prepared for this latest (and final?) makeover.

Chapter 75:
Meeting Doc Fraser
Before the Hysterectomy

A sneak peek into menopause

After saying our hellos and sharing a hug, we got right down to the business at hand– my internal nether regions. Doc Fraser had done a ton of research on the BRCA 1 genetic mutation and was full of helpful information. I admit to feeling like an inconsiderate idiot when he first told me of his preparation for our meeting. Last time I had seen him, we were both under the impression that he would be performing my surgery. Since then, Dr. Tozer had set me up to meet with a surgeon at Henderson. Hmm, I sure wish I had thought to call and let Dr. Fraser know about that minor change of plans. Duh.

In any case, it was extremely reassuring to know that he was looking out for my best interest (not that I had doubted that) and that he was fully informed and able to talk to me about the realities of what I was about to experience. It is a relatively recent discovery, this BRCA 1 (and BRCA 2) thing, so the research, I'm sure, is not entirely consistent (is any research ever completely consistent?).

One thing seems to be recommended time and time again, and that is for women in my situation to do exactly what all of my medical professionals had advised me to do. It was very comforting to be reassured once again that I was doing the right thing. There was no decision to be made, as far as I was concerned. The only question was how quickly I could get in and out of that OR. Again.

I left Dr. Fraser's office feeling good about my upcoming "makeover". He had spent some time educating me on what I could expect post-surgery. Surgical menopause; the immediate cessation of the production of estrogen that had been, up until then, available in hearty portions thanks to two healthy ovaries. How important could estrogen really be? Quite, as it turns out. Damn.

At the ripe old age of 33 (I had enjoyed the celebration of my thirty-third birthday on January 10th and did not share many of my friend's pessimism around the whole "getting older" thing. At this point, getting older was my number one goal, so every year I age from now on, you will hear me hollering it from the rooftops!), I would be facing rapid mood swings (which, according to Jeff, would not be a noticeable change), hot flushes and flashes, vaginal dryness, painful intercourse, increased risk of osteoporosis, memory loss, sleep difficulties and so much more. Soon I would be so hot (literally) that Jeff would hardly be able to stand it (also literally).

Chapter 76:
Meeting My Gynecological Oncologist

Nothing funny about that

Next appointment: Juravinski Cancer Centre; Clinic A. Wow. I was venturing into new territory yet again. I was not heading to the safety of my usual Clinic D appointment, but into the scary waters of Gyne-Oncology. Shiver.

Oddly, I had seriously adopted breast cancer as "my cancer". I had learned as much as I could about it and arrived at a mental place of accepting it, understanding it as much as possible in my position and no longer fearing the trips to Juravinski. I felt safe going to Dr. Tozer's clinic.

Clinic A, on the other hand, freaked me out in a big way. It was simply the unknown. I had once felt that way about Clinic D, too. That seemed like a million years ago. Still, as I drove myself to Hamilton to meet my new surgeon, I confess to having had butterflies in my stomach. I knew it would all work out fine and that Dr. Tozer would not have sent me into the hands of anyone but the best. I just had to get in there and get on with it.

After signing in at the reception desk of Clinic A, and a short wait that I spent faking my way through my latest Oprah pick, I was called by a nurse who led me down a hallway. Ah, that hallway was familiar. I had flashbacks to receiving the results of my genetic testing in a little room somewhere around there. Thank God that was over, at least. I wasn't here to receive news, only to discuss my surgical options with an expert.

I spoke to a nurse who asked me some basic questions for my chart. She then pulled out a clean gown and asked me to strip down below the waist. *Below* the waist? Oh right, it was not a breast thing this time. Freaky. Not as much of a relief as I had imagined to be done with "breast things".

I sat uncomfortably on the examining table admiring my freshly shaven legs, glad to have included my bikini area in the preparations for this particular meeting. In walked my new gyne-oncologist. She introduced herself and we spoke about my medical history. She explained that there were different surgical options for me to consider and that she'd like to examine me first before discussing them in too much detail. After an internal exam she would know better what options applied to me.

That sounded reasonable, all except the internal exam part. It was too late to run screaming so I sucked it up and took yet another one for the team. I will say very little about the exam itself. Some things are better left to the imagination. I will say, however, that upon completion of the aforementioned exam, my soon-to-be surgeon left the room and gave me some time to get dressed. I may have taken a moment or two to rock in the fetal position and then I got it together. I was clothed and relatively calm by the time she returned.

Sitting on her rolling chair at the end of the exam table, the Doc looked directly into my eyes and asked me, and I quote, "Marcie, is anyone here with you today?" Again, the voices were screaming in my head. "Why? What's wrong? What did you find in there?" I asked her in terror. "Oh, nothing. It's just that sometimes people bring others here with them to listen to their surgical options. I didn't want to begin if there was someone else you wanted to get from the waiting room first".

Oh. OK. Maybe on my way out I'll drop a little note in the suggestion box: No one in a lab coat should *ever* ask anyone who has a previous history of any kind of cancer (or anyone who doesn't yet but fears bad news) "Is anyone here with you today?"

The only other time in my life I've heard a question like that was when the Breast Lady called me after my core biopsy, and we all know how that conversation went. Whenever things look fine, the very first thing out of any medical professional's mouth ought to be "Everything looks fine". Anything said after that will be much more well received. Just a suggestion.

Once my heart rate slowed down and the voices hushed to a whisper, I was ready to hear my surgical options. There appeared to be no reason why my surgery could not be done laparoscopically, which was amazing news. Instead of a big abdominal incision I would only have three tiny laparoscope holes. I could deal with that.

My uterus would be removed vaginally (after delivering two babies that way, how bad could "delivering" a uterus be?). My recovery time would be minimal and the procedure should be virtually pain-free. Free is always a good thing, especially where pain is concerned.

I was pleased with our consultation, elated that my doctor agreed to go ahead and book the complete deal. All things removable would be removed "down there" and my risk of ovarian and related cancers would drop in a big way. Clearly, this surgeon knew what she was talking about, had lots of experience and was confident that all would be fine. I trusted her 100 percent.

What choice did I really have?

Chapter 77:
Megan Rose Noye's Big Idea

She's sugar and spice and everything pink

It was around the time that my hysterectomy was being scheduled that I got a call from the Maritimes. It was Tanya and she was excited about something. I couldn't wait to hear what it was.

As it turned out, her daughter, Megan, had been spending a lot of time thinking about her birthday and what kind of party she'd like to have. She would be turning seven on April 17th and was right into planning the details of the event.

Megan is a very mature girl and has always seemed older than her age. I remember her sitting on our kitchen floor one summer while on vacation. She couldn't have been much more than three, if that. She was playing with the alphabet fridge magnets and I was quietly watching her.

I was awestruck as I realized that she was not just playing around randomly, moving letters from one side of the fridge to the other. She was spelling words. Real words. Cat. Dog. Megan. Up. It. Holy crap. OK, she didn't spell that last one, but it's what I was thinking as I observed her.

So it was no surprise to me that Megan, at six years old going on 16, had a big idea. She, of course, been kept informed in an age-appropriate way, of what I had been going through. She knew about my breast cancer. She knew about my surgeries. She understood much more than Bryn did. In fact, I am still convinced that she understood much more than any person her age would typically understand.

This year, Megan had decided all on her own that she would like to have a "Think Pink" party in my honour. She would ask for everyone invited to come wearing pink from head to toe. Instead of gifts for her, she would ask that donations be made in my name to the Canadian Breast Cancer Foundation. How beyond amazing is that? She was excited to do this. No one was forcing her hand, that's for sure.

I listened as Tanya choked back tears. There is nothing better than pure motherly pride. Her daughter was clearly turning out OK. As far as parenting goes, I think I'll start taking notes from Tanya and Mike. Wow.

Of course I received an invitation to the party, even though it was going to take place right around my surgery date. I would have given everything to have been there. I secretly and regularly fantasized about showing up unexpectedly and being in the brightest, pinkest outfit ever seen. Megan deserved that. I still regret not being able to Think Pink with Megan and her family and friends.

The only thing I could do to show my love, appreciation and, hey, let's face it, adoration, was to hit the mall. Big time. If that little girl thought she was not going to get any birthday presents this year, she was mistaken!

Have you ever gone in search of pink clothes and accessories for little girls? They grow on trees. The problem was not finding a pink gift for Megan, but deciding what to buy and what to leave behind. If I'd have had a money tree that day, the possibilities would've been endless.

I eventually decided on a pink outfit, including fancy shiny shoes, and a big bag to go with it. A soft fuzzy pink teddy bear. A pink watch. All manner of pink goodies. But the best part, in my opinion, was the little pink angel that goes on a window. I had quickly decided it was perfect, not only because the proceeds of the purchase would go directly to breast cancer research, but because Megan was my little earth angel, praying for me and taking me under her wing.

I forced myself to leave the mall, loaded up the trunk with pink girlie things, and headed straight for the Post Office. I put the loot into a big box, had it weighed, addressed it and sent it on its way. I couldn't wait until it arrived in Halifax. I knew it would get there in time for the big party. I hoped Megan would love the gifts. I hoped that she would somehow be able to feel my love for her all the way across the miles as she opened the box. I prayed hard that somehow, someday, I would be able to truly show that amazing little girl how thankful I really was. Oh, and I also secretly hoped she'd choose the outfit *I* bought her to wear at her party. (She did.)

Chapter 78:
The Hysterectomy

Always go with your gut feeling

I have many memories about the hysterectomy/salpingo-oopherectomy surgeries, most of which I will save you the horror of reading about. I *will* tell you that I arrived at Henderson Hospital on the day of my surgery feeling slightly nervous but ready to have my procedures. I had followed the pre-op instructions carefully the day before. My bowels were prepped (don't ask). My legs were shaved. I was hungry. I've heard that some people actually lose their appetites when they are nervous. Me, not so much.

I went through very much the same routine as with the previous surgeries, and it was reassuring that this hospital, although I'd never been operated on there, seemed to follow the same general preparatory steps that I had become used to at Guelph General.

When the time came for me to be moved to the pre-op waiting room, I knew that things would soon be underway. An anesthetist came to my bedside and verified some information on my chart. He asked me what my plan was for pain relief. I asked him what my options were. This guy had done his homework. He was well aware of my recent medical history and was very intent on making this surgery as pain-free and bearable as possible. Needless to say, I bonded with him immediately.

As it turned out, after coming out of the general anesthesia, one option for pain relief was going to be the use of a pain pump. The thought of pumping morphine into my body actually made me gag. No, a night of post-surgical barfing was not my first choice. I had already crossed that off my "to-do" list.

My second option, and clearly the only one that made any sense to me as I lay there awaiting a major surgery, was to go with a spinal epidural. Although my recovery would be much easier and less painful if my surgeon was able to remove my ovaries and fallopian tubes by laparoscopy, the anesthetist explained that there was still a chance that the doctor would end up having to open up my abdominal area instead. There was no way to be certain until she went in there and got started. An epidural would allow me to recover in a pain-free fashion if that were the case. One large needle in my spine, please. Where do you need me to sign for that?

The decision was easy; given that option A (the morphine pump) really wasn't a viable option at all. The anesthetist and I discussed how the spinal epidural would work. I told him that I was kind of an expert as far as that procedure went, what with the births of my daughters and all. He promised me that while having an epidural would definitely take away all feeling from the waist down, it would in no way increase my chances of waking up with a newborn baby in my arms. Phew. That would've been a deal-breaker.

Next, while the anesthetist was off preparing for my epidural, the Big Boss approached my bedside. It was a relief to see my gyne-oncologist in her operating room gear, clearly ready to go ahead with my surgery. She told me that she was nearly ready for me and that this surgery, if she did her job well, would be painless. I explained that I would be having an epidural before my general anesthetic, so I would be pain free upon awaking from surgery (even if she didn't do her job well. Don't worry. I didn't say that part out loud).

Now, here's an awkward situation. The surgeon told me that I absolutely did not need an epidural and that having one would only slow down my recovery and keep me in the hospital longer. It wasn't necessary, so never mind. She was the one about to start removing my innards one way or another, so I felt it was of paramount importance that I disagree with her very politely.

As any woman who has been through health problems and who has had to learn to stand up for herself when there is a medical decision to be made about her body would do, I blamed someone else. I told her that my anesthetist really encouraged me to go with the epidural, in case the laparoscopic procedure didn't work out for some reason. He was very confident that this was the way to go for me. Right, but there was no reason to believe that the plan to use laparoscopy wouldn't work. None. Again, we were at a standoff.

The surgeon left my bedside, turning and walking directly into the operating room. I hoped she didn't have the authority to fire the anesthetist. I really did want that epidural. By the time I was wheeled into the OR, I had forgotten all about the whole pain-relief thing. I was just happy to be in that room, one step closer to yet another sweet narcotic-induced blackout.

My people, my team, were assembled around me. Like a well-oiled machine, I thought. My anesthetist/new best friend asked me to sit up and open my gown (from the back, this time). He needed to sterilize my back before putting the needle in. At that moment, the surgeon asked him what he was doing. Uh oh.

Let's just say that there was a "professional difference of opinion" involved. My anesthetist held his ground like a pro and my surgeon was not happy about it. The good news: I got the epidural in the end. The bad news: I had an angry surgeon about to open me up.

Panic. Terror. Darkness.

The most important thing to know about the hysterectomy experience was that my gyne-oncologist did more than a good job. She did an amazing job. It baffles me to this day that she was able to do all that she did with only three tiny little holes (and one larger one), barely noticeable. The laparoscopic approach worked like a charm and I soon found myself awake, shaking but relieved and completely pain free. Unfortunately, I couldn't tell if I was pain-free because the surgery had been done so well or because of the spinal epidural. Either way, I felt like a million dollars.

I have to admit that I am grateful to the anesthetist for sticking up for me *and* I am thankful to the surgeon for also doing what she felt was best for me. When you think about it, there are definitely worse problems to have than two qualified, highly respected doctors arguing over how to best take care of you while you are in the hospital.

I ended up spending two nights in the hospital (mainly because the epidural had slowed down my recovery by approximately one night). OK, score one for the surgeon. Still, I wouldn't have traded my epidural for anything, not even a ticket out of there 24 hours earlier. Score one for the anesthetist. Let's just call it even and move on.

On the first morning after the surgery, I received a visit from my surgeon. She sat on the end of my bed and told me that everything had gone very well the day before. What a relief I felt for a second. Why couldn't she have just gotten up and left my room at that point? She *had* noticed, however, that my uterus had been extremely soft when she removed it. I, of course, understood immediately that by "extremely soft" she actually meant "softer than normal". I panicked, asking her what that meant. What could be the cause of an overly soft uterus? Was it a sign of some reproductive cancer? To put my fears at rest, my gyne-oncologist looked directly into my eyes and explained that my uterus was probably so soft because I was still breastfeeding. I kid you not.

Hmmm. No, I wasn't *still* breastfeeding. I understand that the body parts above my waist are not really her specialty. I get that she had been focusing her work on the lower half of my body (which is good, because everything I needed her to remove was down there). Still, I desperately wanted to holler at her, "Look up! *No breasts up here*". No breastfeeding going on. In that case, she informed me, we'd just have to wait for the pathology report to come back in a couple of weeks. *Then* she left my room. It was probably nothing. When had I heard that before? Sigh.

After my two-night stay, I called Jeff to come pick me up. I got myself changed. I packed my bags. I said my goodbyes to the nurses who had taken such good care of me. It is true that even though the hysterectomy experience was certainly riddled with ups and downs, the bottom line is that, having been through one more major surgery, I walked out of that hospital without pain in my belly. Isn't that something?

Chapter 79:
The Pathology Report

Extra! Extra! Read all about it!

You will notice that I have not devoted a chapter to my at-home recovery from the hysterectomy surgery. That is because, for all intents and purposes, there was no recovery. Technically I had a lot to recover from, but it was painless and did not get me down the way the previous surgeries and treatments had. Really, it was just enough of a recovery for me to truly need some help, but not enough of one that I actually needed help with every single aspect of my life. I moved a bit more slowly than normal, I wasn't able to lug the kids around as I used to, but otherwise I was feeling relatively well.

Except for the whole, "Let's just wait and see why your uterus isn't like the others" thing. Oh boy - Jeff and I found ourselves awaiting yet another big phone call. I have never thought of myself as overly dramatic (I don't know if others have ever thought of me that way. It's best not to ask that type of question.) but I admit to allowing myself to obsess about the possibility of a problem with my uterus. Once you have received bad news, *really bad* news, it is much easier to see the glass as half empty the next time around. In my mind, a soft uterus was a death sentence.

Needless to say, by the time "the phone call" from my surgeon came, I had already convinced myself (and my husband) that the news would be bad. I had undergone a surgery for preventative measures, but it had been too late. I could feel it. I was screwed. My uterus would be the end of me after all. How ironic that my breasts weren't going to be to blame for my untimely demise. Maybe if I'd had a more difficult physical recovery, I'd have had less mental energy to play the "get yourself into a hysterical state and stay that way" game. Damn that laparoscope.

The phone rang. I grabbed it. I heard a very serious female voice ask for me. "Speaking". It was my surgeon. She said, and I loosely quote, "The *good* news is that your pathology report looks fine. I also did a wash with a dye that indicated no disease on any organs inside your abdominal area". Silence. Silence. Silence. OK, so what's the *bad* news? "Oh, that's great to hear. Is that everything, then?" "Yes, unless you have any questions for me". Well, just one: Are you trying to mess with my head? Don't say, "the *good* news is ..." unless it is going to be followed by "but the *bad* news is ..."

Hey, I'm not complaining about the fact that my body was cancer-free. Just about the fact that until 10 seconds earlier I had truly believed that I was about to find out I was dying. "No, no questions." Let's not go there. "Thank you so much, doctor. Thank you. Thank you. Thank you." Click. Silence. Then, sobbing. Thank you, God.

I received that joyous news of a clean bill of health exactly two days before the one-year anniversary of my breast cancer diagnosis. So, there I sat, one year later, crying hysterically after a phone conversation with a surgeon. Only this time, I was crying tears of utter relief, joy, and happiness. Victory. I had my health. I was cancer-free. I was a breast cancer *survivor*. Sweet.

For someone who isn't a fan of talking on the phone, I sure spent a lot of time calling friends and family after my big news. I was well. I wanted to shout it from the rooftop. I did it! We had all done it; me, my husband, my kids, my family, my friends, my doctors. Together. Now it was time to celebrate by living my life to its fullest. Every day. Starting now. Poutine, anyone?

Chapter 80:
Surgical Menopause

One hot mama

I continued recovering from my latest surgery and, as far as recoveries go, it was not too bad. I was careful not to do too much or walk too quickly, but I didn't take much pain medication once I got home from the hospital. I still held Dana (a no-no according to the info sheet I was sent home with), but didn't lug her around all over the place as I would have normally. Bryn could still sit on my lap gently and snuggle with me. So, from a mom's perspective, I was doing OK.

There were, however, certain changes that were noticeable pretty much immediately. I had automatically reserved my room with a fireplace at the Roehampton B&B so was spending my first nights post-surgery away from home (well, at my home away from home, anyway).

As I mentioned earlier, I didn't feel too awful pain-wise at that time, but I was exhausted and could definitely feel my body (and mind) struggling to make sense of the newest version of me, inside and out. It is mind-boggling that a person, a body, could go through so much in such a short period of time. After each trauma, I felt as though there had not been enough time to fully recover before the next one was necessary.

Even though Dr. Fraser had warned me about menopause and it's spectrum of symptoms, for me, it falls into the category of "must experience it to understand or believe it". Yes, like childbirth and a cancer diagnosis, there are no words to adequately describe what menopause really means or how it affects all aspects of daily life. At least that was my experience. Still is.

I recall the exact moment that menopause came out to play. I had been fast asleep (medically assisted, as I was still unable to fall asleep or stay asleep for any length of time on my own) in my cozy bed at The Roehamptons. I awoke literally in a hot flash from hell. I frantically threw off the covers, tore off my pyjamas and stood, heart pounding, for what seemed like forever. I knew, without any past experience, that I had just had a hot flash. Brutal.

That first hot flash turned out to be one of many, varying in duration and intensity. For someone who already had trouble sleeping, the onslaught of sometimes four or five hot flashes each night was disheartening at best (infuriating at worst, but that might be my mood swings talking). I learned quickly to layer my clothes (especially at night when the hot flashes were much more frequent and often more intense), with light camisoles or tank tops under button-down or zip-up shirts for easy peeling. I've never been a fan of sleeping in my birthday suit but it was very tempting in the early days of menopause.

In addition to the hot flashes, I noticed, over time, that there were mood swings and then there were *mood swings*. I longed for the good old days when a mood swing was related to PMS. Those ones were fun compared to the new and mighty ones. I swear to you that there were times when my ups and downs even terrified me (so I don't have to tell you how fun I was to live with at that point).

One of the problems with the menopause mood swings, I found, was that there was no "x" on the calendar marking an end to them. No menstruation. No PMS leading up to menstruation. Just hot flashes and mood swings as far as the eye could see. Bad news for my whole family. Jeff could no longer cling to the knowledge that on a particular date, his misery would come to an end, until the next month, at least.

To look on the bright side, my highs and lows certainly made our marriage more spontaneous. Spontaneous fits of hysterical sobbing. Spontaneous demands for a divorce because he forgot to add eggs to the grocery list on the fridge after using the last one. Spontaneous talks about "us" and what he was "thinking". Trust me; he had the sense to know enough to *never* tell me what he was actually thinking at those moments. So among its many other "benefits", menopause certainly played a role in spicing up our marriage.

Chapter 81:
Chemo-Induced Memory Loss

Did I tell you this already?

Along with the challenges of instantly becoming a post-menopausal woman, add in the loss of memory in a big way. You've likely heard the expression, "She'd lose her head if it weren't attached". That was me. And it was a really good thing my head *was* attached (not that I found the brain in my head to be terribly helpful much of the time).

At the time of my recovery from the hysterectomy, when I was only beginning to understand the massive life change that necessarily accompanied being a 33 year-old woman trapped in a 60 year-old woman's body, I was still quite concerned about the severity of the memory loss I had experienced as a side effect of chemotherapy. Dr. Tozer (and all the literature I had read on the topic) assured me that it was perfectly normal to notice memory loss post-chemo and that, thankfully, this side effect would be temporary. For many women, the dulling of the gray matter (affectionately referred to as "chemo fog") often proved to be relatively short-lived.

However, you may have noticed a trend in the direction of me *not* being just like the many women for whom things run smoothly? As far as my brain went, it appeared that I had lost more cells than I could afford to in order to maintain even the appearance of being "fine". Yes, in my case, the brain damage was quite severe and quite frustrating (to myself as well as to those poor souls who were regularly forced to tell me the same thing over and over again ad nauseam).

I learned to use certain memory tricks, such as writing everything on sticky notes. I also carried a couple of pens (in case one ran out unexpectedly or I forgot where I put one) and kept a little coil notebook in my purse and coat pocket at all times. Anything that did not get written down immediately ceased to have happened or existed in my world. It was really that bad.

Can you picture the look on my face upon learning from Dr. Fraser at our pre-hysterectomy meeting that one of the very common side effects of menopause was memory loss? That was going to be a problem for me (or at least it would have been, had I not forgotten even meeting with Dr. Fraser by the time I left his office and walked to my car).

I figured that, with my luck, on day one of my new menopausal life, I would look into my daughters' eyes and find something very familiar about them. I feared I would actually cease to recognize my own offspring if I suffered any further memory loss! The very thought of living with a worse memory really ticked me off in a big, big way. I just wanted to scream with intense rage at the unfairness of it all (unless it was just the mood swings of menopause getting to me).

At that point, I was guessing that dementia might be the straw that broke my patient husband's back in our marriage. What *was* his name again? He would have been fully justified, at that time, in running off with an energetic senior citizen. How could I compete with that?

Sure enough, as time went by, the loss of memory became very apparent in all aspects of my daily life. I kid you not when I say that it came to a point when I was literally unable to remember what I had just been doing, to whom I had been speaking on the phone for the past hour and, when driving down the road, where it was I had been going. Several times I had to pull over, close my eyes, and try desperately to remember where I was headed. The harder I tried, the more I would panic. The more I panicked, the less likely it became that I would remember. There were even times when I turned the car around and drove home in tears. Honestly, sometimes I never did remember where I had been going.

On the rare occasion that I would actually remember where I was heading, there was yet another roadblock. I could picture the end destination but not the way to get there. My brain, it seemed, had lost its inner maps. Simple routes became mazes. I would get lost on my way from my house to the mall. I would drive slowly, desperately looking around for landmarks, memory triggers. Sometimes it would all come back to me as quickly as it had left, but other times I drove around aimlessly before admitting defeat and returning home.

While there is certainly a very humorous element to my tales of memory loss, the reality on a day-to-day basis was, at times, unbearable. I recall sitting on the couch crying in frustration. Crying in fear. What if my memory never returned to normal? I was embarrassed and ashamed that I had actually been reduced to the low point of taking Bryn with me to run errands and telling her in advance where we would be going and what we would be buying at each stop. Then, as would inevitably happen at some point in our travels, I would draw a blank and have to ask her where we were going. She would happily remind me, saying "silly mommy" and we would continue on our way.

I was unable to come up with a reasonable explanation for returning home without making any of our planned stops on those days when my memory refused to produce a map with which I could find my way to a desired location. I remember making up little excuses such as, "Oh dear, I forgot my wallet at home. That's OK, we'll go to the bank later", or "I have an idea, why don't we go home to play for a while and we can stop at the bakery after we pick daddy up from work?" To a four-year-old little girl, returning home to play Uno instead of waiting in a line up at the bank was a dream come true. Thankfully, she was still too young to realize what was really going on.

Luckily, at least some of the more severe memory lapses seemed to fade over time, although never to the point that I have felt "like my old self". I still lose things, spend way too much time retracing my steps in an effort to find my keys, my purse, my children. Okay, I've never lost my children. I may have tried but they're way too smart.

I also feel overwhelmed easily, stop mid-sentence with no clue what I was saying, and have come to accept that my old brain is not what it used to be. I suppose it would be expecting a lot to put my body and mind through a chemical war against cancer cells without suffering any side effects. Still, I am not without hope that my memory will someday return to what it once was. One day at a time. In the meantime, I will use the "chemo card" whenever I need to, whether that is really the problem or not!

Chapter 82:
Long Term Disability

Show me the money!

As Jeff and I continued to adjust to the "new normal", the ebb and flow of our daily lives since cancer's unwelcome entrance into our lives, we were forced to establish a new relationship with money. Up until that point, we had both always worked hard, made enough money to live comfortably and enjoy many perks and treats. We had been financially blessed in the same way that we had been blessed with our health and loved ones.

Before my cancer diagnosis, Jeff and I were getting psyched up to live a bit leaner. I was going to be on maternity leave, making significantly less money than what we were accustomed to and we would have two children to feed and clothe. Still, we knew we would be fine, and any sacrifices we had to make for our girls would be well worth it.

Needless to say, we had barely wrapped our heads around the new "cheap bastard budget", as Jeff so lovingly called it, when we learned that not only would I not be on maternity leave, but that I would be on long term disability pay instead. We were in uncharted financial territory. Neither one of us had ever really looked into how our LTD benefits worked. Again, this was an area we had been lucky enough to never need before.

Our heads were spinning with change. I have a history of fearing change, so this was quite traumatic on many levels. There was necessary paperwork to complete. There were insurance agents to speak to, questions to answer and an unending stream of voice mail messages to return. If you will recall, using the telephone was never one of my strong suits. Poor insurance company!

Thankfully, we were not entirely on our own. My principal at Brant Avenue Public School was able to help me initially navigate the paperwork to be handed in at the school board level. I got to know the team of supportive board employees who were working on my claim.

Lynda McDougall, my teachers' union VP, also went out of her way to walk me through all stages of the process. She was extremely compassionate and spoke in terms that I could easily understand (and whenever I didn't understand, it was definitely the chemo fog to blame, not Lynda's choice of words!). Turned out I was not the first ever board employee to need disability assistance!

As with any bureaucracy, no matter how many people there were who genuinely wanted to help me through the financial mess of "sick leave", it still felt as if each little step forward led to several giant steps back.

Part of the problem was that there were different people I needed to call to speak to depending on the question. There were a lot of answering machines (how rude of someone not to answer their phone ...) requiring detailed messages. It wasn't so bad actually leaving the messages, when I remembered to do so (which was rarely), but it was pure hell having so many people call me back! Not many days went by without my phone ringing off the hook. I hated that.

Each time someone would call me back, I'd have to rack my brain to remember exactly why I had left the message in the first place. It was all very confusing and irritating, to be honest. I remember crying to Jeff on several occasions. There just had to be an easier way.

The worst, most horribly stressful thing that happened while I was on LTD began with yet another bloody phone call. I can't remember whom I spoke to, but it was someone calling from the payroll department of the school board. By some crazy fluke of nature, there had been an error and the school board had accidentally been paying me for several months when I was not supposed to be receiving pay. Interesting. Did I not wonder why I was getting pay stubs from work while off work?

No. Because I hadn't received any pay stubs from work. I *was* in a chemo fog but I had not gone *blind*. I did look at my mail regularly and there had been no correspondence from work. Didn't I know that the board had begun using electronic pay stubs instead of paper ones? No again. I hadn't been using my work e-mail because I was not working! I was ill. So when I finally looked at my old work e-mails, sure enough there were several electronic paystubs dating back to the first school week in September.

You may wonder how I, we, had not noticed an overpayment going into our bank account. We just didn't. It's that simple. We had no clue what the hell was going on with our finances or who was supposed to be paying me what and when, so the fact that we were not struggling more financially seemed like a bright light in an otherwise dark tunnel. Trust me, worrying about my life and caring for our children at that time in our lives pretty much made everything else take a back burner. We chose our battles and had no choice but to let other people do their jobs. We figured I had filled in all of the necessary paperwork. My part was done. It was up to the board and the government to do the rest.

My mom used to say that to assume "made an ass out of u and me". Get it? Assume? Well, once again, she was right. Our assumption that our finances were running along smoothly and our less than eagle-eyed approach to minding our money at that time led to a huge debt. Yup. It was the school board's error but I would be the one to fix it. Okay, Jeff would be the one to fix it. He was the one with the job, after all! Literally thousands of dollars that we did not have were owed to the school board. I did indeed feel like an ass.

The moral of the story is: if it seems as though you have more money than you're supposed to have in any given situation, then you probably do. At least have the sense to look into it and make sure an error has not occurred that will cost you later on. If you don't, you too will wind up feeling like an ass. A broke ass.

Chapter 83:
The View from a Stick

What a difference a year makes

As I type this chapter, I look back on more than a year of life with breast cancer. Life battling breast cancer. Fearing breast cancer. Accepting breast cancer. Living well with breast cancer. Beating breast cancer.

Not long ago, my neighbour and I were visiting while our kids played on their bikes between the two houses. She mentioned to me that a woman a few doors down had just had a mastectomy and was awaiting news on her treatment plan. She was a mother of two young sons, one seven and one 14, and the wife of a wonderfully supportive man whose life had just fallen apart with the news. She did not have much family or many friends in the country to help her. She was terrified and alone.

I couldn't wait to meet my neighbour; this sister/survivor/friend. I had learned that you don't need to know someone personally to feel an instant connection to him or her. Cancer brings people together, that's for sure.

As I knocked on her door that same week, I marvelled at the fact that I was, only one year after my own devastating diagnosis, in a position to help and comfort a woman with breast cancer. I could tell her she would get through this. I could tell her that I understood her fear and pain. I could tell her all that I had learned. I could help.

When we met face to face, her relief was palpable. She needed to know someone who had been in her shoes and lived to tell, as I had needed my Pink Ladies so many months ago. We became fast friends, supporting each other, laughing and crying together. I took her to her chemotherapy treatments a couple of times. I sat and listened when she needed to vent. I gave her my shoulder to cry on. I felt very strong and blessed to be in a position to give her comfort.

I was glad to be her Pink Lady. I wore the title proudly and the symbolic passing of the breast cancer torch that had taken place between us was not lost on me. Over time, I slipped slowly into the background and allowed her to stretch her wings and fly on her own. I had fought my battle. I could not fight hers, as much as I wanted to try. This was *her* story, not my own.

I suppose we all have tests of faith. Tests of strength. For me, it was breast cancer. For you, it may be something altogether different. Regardless of the details, it is human to suffer along life's journey. Here's what I have come up with to get me through the rest of life's ups and downs (I am not naïve enough to believe that breast cancer was my one and only hurdle in this lifetime).

The strength of the human spirit is nothing short of miraculous. If someone had told me even two years ago that I would be diagnosed with breast cancer while pregnant, undergo a lumpectomy, bilateral mastectomies, six months of aggressive chemotherapy treatments, receive results of genetic testing that would prove the existence in my body of a mutation predisposing me (and, possibly my children, someday) to breast cancer all followed up by the preventative removal of my uterus, cervix, fallopian tubes and ovaries, I would have either laughed in their face or run screaming, or both. Instead, it all happened and it was all do-able. Crappy but do-able.

To read my own story, I am guessing that I will need to have large amounts of alcohol in my system. Believe me, I am well aware of the "holy crap" factor that accompanies my tale. When people hear my story for the first time, I can see the disbelief in their eyes. Sometimes *I* cannot believe that it was real. And then I look down. At my chest. At my scars. It was real. Very real.

Here's the thing: the day before my cancer diagnosis I was Marcie Nolan (or Marcie Adams, if you were my doctor). I had a loving family, a beautiful daughter and one on the way, the best husband a girl could dream of, friends to support and encourage me, a love of God and my health. My body was beautiful. I had great breasts. Two, to be exact. And many healthy internal organs.

Today, I am still Marcie Nolan (or Marcie Adams, if you're one of my many doctors). I have a loving family, two beautiful daughters, the best husband a girl could dream of, friends to support and encourage me, a love of God and my health. My body is beautiful. I may be short two breasts and the reproductive organs that had made it possible to bring my two babies into the world, but to be honest, I haven't missed them all that much.

To me, my flat, scarred chest is a symbol of strength. I am definitely not my body alone. I am a complete package. A spirit, mind and body. An altered but healthy, fully functioning body is worth more to me now than the perkiest pair of breasts I could buy. And, hey, you *can* buy breasts, you know. I've never heard of a person buying a large bottle of "perfect health". It's all we really want. It's all we really need. Without it, I have learned, life is hard, regardless of your breast size.

I like to think of myself as "the new beautiful". I now possess the kind of beauty that I plan to teach my children (and anyone else who will listen) to appreciate and value far more than the style of their hair or the labels on their clothes. Lying in a hospital bed in the same blue "gown" as every other patient in the building, suddenly what brand of jeans I owned ceased to matter. As I went out into the world a bald young mother undergoing chemotherapy, it became crystal clear how little a role my hair had in defining me as a person. Talk about being forced to look within!

So, I have said goodbye to my breasts. I have said goodbye to my reproductive organs. I will say goodbye to any part of me that is unhealthy and damaging to my quality of life on earth. Let them remove what they may. Just let them keep me well.

And so, when, someday, I find myself facing physical or emotional adversity (as is bound to happen as long as I am human and alive), I will look back upon this time and know that I will be OK. I will draw strength from the successes of my past. I can truly say that if, one day, I find myself in the terrifying position of having lost additional parts of my physical self to a disease that counts me as only one of so many in its clutches, then I plan to hold my head up high. I understand now in a new and deeper way that I could lose so much more and still be me.

I have also learned from my breast cancer journey that it is easier to face the ugliness of the unknown head-on; to stare it down bravely rather than to let my fear of the future swallow me whole. I have faced my worst fears for the future many times in my mind's eye and have smiled widely at what I have allowed myself to see: I *may* have a recurrence. I *may* lose more parts. I *may* undergo further surgeries. I *may* find myself dependent upon more medical professionals to help me along the way. I *may* once again need to lean on my family and friends for support and strength. And then again, I *may* not.

And yet, *even* if the day comes that I am physically nothing more than a head on a stick, having said good-bye to who I am at this moment in time (to this new and improved cancer-surviving me), I have made a promise to myself that I will be a head on a stick with a smile on my face. I will hold my head up high. I will enjoy my days as long as I have life in me.

At the end of the day, who can say with any certainty how a life will unfold? The lesson here, for me, at least, is to live today with the knowledge that this day is precious. No other day will be exactly like this one. *Today* matters more than I ever realized before cancer. What happened yesterday cannot be changed. What happens tomorrow will reveal itself tomorrow, so why waste today living in the past or the future? The present is right here waiting to be noticed and enjoyed.

I prefer to focus my energy now on the things I have gained. I have cut my losses (no pun intended) and can thank my cancer experience for bringing many positive changes to my life. I could write another whole book on the ups and downs of my world as a cancer survivor; as Marcie Nolan. Perhaps I will.

Epilogue

This is not the end

Today Bryn is a going concern. I alternate between wanting to squeeze her, kiss her and hold her forever and wanting to send her to her Auntie Bug's house until she's 20. I hear from my friends that Bryn is behaving just like the rest of the little terrors, er, I mean darlings.

Bryn knows her mind. She is confident. She is bright. She is curious. She is a good friend to others. She is verbally advanced but doesn't know it, she can dress up in a knight's armour, Daniel Boon cap and high-heeled shoes and *totally* make it work, *and* she makes me proud every moment of every day. Even when it is all I can do to keep from putting a "Please look after this child." sign around her little neck and dropping her off on Papa and Nana's front porch, I am forever amazed at the wondrous person that she has become.

Dana, our angel baby, is another girl on the go. She is a child who sees no limits. Nothing in this world is in her way (not for long, anyway). She is perfectly well adjusted and seems not to remember a life other than the one she is living with us today. I envy her that ignorance at times!

Dana is the picture of perfection in her lavender-framed spectacles and her impish smile. In her face I see so much life, so much strength, so much personality and an intricate mix of my mom, my dad and myself. On the other hand, she is unique in the world. I could not have designed a more interesting, loving, perfect little girl if I had tried.

Judging from the look and character of each of my daughter's, I am pleased to note that not *all* of my genes were faulty. I will give a touch of credit to Jeff's part in their creation; however I prefer to see their best qualities as coming directly from *my* people. It is the tantrums, food-flinging, name-calling and gas that I attribute to the Nolan genes!

I am also happy to report that the entire cancer experience is only one small part of my life as a mother and Jeff's life as a father. To our children, we are still parents first and everything else second. We are still mommy and daddy, and that is exactly who we want to be.

An amazing fact (even to me) is that, as an offshoot of my recent experiences with poor health, I have made the commitment to treat myself as well as I treat my children. For so long, I would spend time every morning preparing a healthy, well-balanced and tasty breakfast for my girls. "There is no more important meal in the day", I reminded them regularly. After all, a healthy breakfast is where you will get your energy to enjoy the day, right? "Now run along and play so mommy can drink her double double while it's still hot".

Now I sit with my kids (most days) and enjoy the same nutritious breakfast as they do. Knowing that a large coffee does not constitute a complete breakfast is one thing; making the changes to my diet to improve my health is quite another. You'd think the fear of dying or greater chances of a breast cancer recurrence would be motivation enough to eat better for someone with half a brain in her head, wouldn't you? (And I'm pretty sure I still *have* half a brain, if only I could remember where I put it ...) Never underestimate the power of a Tim Hortons coffee.

Seriously, though, I still enjoy a coffee a day, often a home brew with skim milk and a touch of sugar, but after that first coffee I switch to herbal teas and water with lemon. Both were an acquired taste and there are still lots of times when the initial sip or two are forced. I do, in the end, enjoy these drinks and feel good about myself for taking care of my body the way I have always known I should.

In addition to my new breakfast ritual and limited caffeine intake, I have made a great effort to plan meals and snacks more consciously. I am eating far more fruits and veggies than I ever have before. The crazy thing is that I have always loved fruits and veggies. I was just too lazy to wash, dry, peel, cut or prepare them. Ripping open a breakfast bar or having a second large coffee was quicker and easier, and seemed to fill me up as much. In a short period of time, however, I have grown to crave the good stuff. A meal without a salad or some kind of fresh veggie seems incomplete.

Again, let me stress to you that I am doing this in moderation. I have it in me to be a bit extreme and, in the past, I admit to having taken food restriction and dieting past a healthy point. My goal now is very simple: to achieve optimal health and reap the benefits of more energy and better sleep that will accompany such good health (and if my sex life happens to benefit from this lifestyle change then so be it. Wink).

I don't need to swear off cheese (blasphemy!) or chocolate or fries or … mmm, fries … sorry, what was I saying? I only need to add more good stuff to my plate and listen to my body's signals. Turns out you are supposed to stop eating when you are full, even if you haven't finished all the food on your plate yet. Were you aware of that? Man, this new age stuff is all a mystery to me.

Who knows what my life might have been like had I not been diagnosed with breast cancer at such a young age? In the end, it doesn't matter much. I am here now. I am healthy, I am loved and I am happy. In the past, I could never understand it when I heard people say that a cancer diagnosis was the greatest gift they had ever been given. I admit that now, looking back, that doesn't sound like such a crazy thought. I would never have chosen this path for myself. No one would. Yet, I have gained so much; learned so much; lived so much more fully as a result of it having happened. I suppose it was simply meant to be. For better or worse (and I think for better, most days) cancer has touched me. It has changed me. I am who I am today (a survivor), in part, because of my cancer experience.

I am proud that I have survived cancer. I am certain that now I can survive anything.

Afterword

Email from Tanya to Marcie on June 21, 2007, 3:06pm

When I started writing this, it was my intention to cheer you up. I think it actually made me more aware of how important you have been to me in my life. I have been unsure about sending it, but after talking to you today, I feel that I must let you know what you mean to me as best as I can. Like I said earlier, this is absolutely not intended to be an addition to your book, but simply to encourage you to get it out into the world. I hope you like the quotes I picked out for you at the end.

I love you and thank God that you are in my life!

Love,
Tanya xox

We know that trouble is a part of life. If you don't share it, you don't give the people who love you a chance to love you enough. – Unknown

Marcie and I have laughed over nothing and cried over everything. We know everything about each other, good and bad, and never have two people understood each other as we do. To say she is my best friend is truly an understatement. She is my sister; a true kindred spirit.

We met in 1983 when her family moved to Halifax. I remember our first encounter like it was yesterday. I was sitting in art class listening to the art teacher yell while the veins in her blood red face and neck bulged out when the door opened... "Class, this is our new student, Marcie", said our grade four homeroom teacher. Luckily there was an empty seat beside me for this wide eyed girl. She quietly sat down, the door shut, and the art teacher picked up right where she had left off. I saw the terror in Marcie's face, so to comfort her I leaned over. "Don't worry. She does this all the time!" I said. We both smiled and were inseparable from that moment on. Well, almost inseparable.

Two years later came the horrible news; Marcie's family was moving back to Ontario! It felt like someone had reached into my chest and pulled out my heart. How would two twelve year old girls stay in contact and remain best friends from thousands of miles apart?

I'm happy to say we did! Calling each other every moment we could, writing letter after letter, and begging our parents every summer to fly us to see the other. She is the very reason I started working at such a young age. Most fourteen year olds wanted to spend their money on clothes or makeup. Not me! I had long distance phone bills and summertime airfare to save for. Keep in mind that this was before computers were in every home, and no one had ever even heard of text messaging!

Over the years and the distance, somehow our friendship grew stronger and stronger. I can honestly say we have been there for each other through everything; Marcie's mother's sudden passing, our weddings, the birth of our children, and now we can add breast cancer to our long list. I still remember getting that dreadful phone call. "Are you sitting down?" she said in a shaky voice. Then those awful and unforgettable words "breast cancer" came out. After many tears, "what the…", and "oh my God", we said goodbye, totally stunned. A little while later Marcie called to apologize for "dropping a huge bomb" on me like that. She was worried about me and hoped I was okay. Worried about ME!?! Can you imagine? She was just diagnosed with breast cancer and she was worrying about me. You don't get any more thoughtful than that!

Marcie has such a gift for always making whomever she meets feel good about themselves. This book is no exception to that. She has somehow managed to take this horrific experience, turn it into a humorous and uplifting story, and has unselfishly put it out into the world to share with everyone in order to help others overcome their battle.

Although we have had some major changes throughout our lives, I know one thing will remain constant; our friendship. Marcie will always be the person I can complain to, laugh with, cry with, and eat large amounts of cheese with! She holds my heart like no one else can and I am truly blessed just to have known her.

Tanya Noye

Acknowledgements

There are too many wonderful people in my support system to mention every one by name. Thank you to all who made my journey easier along the way.

Special thanks to:

My amazing editors: Linda Lazier, Mary K. Nolan and Shelley Welstead. This book is even better because of you.

My husband, Jeff, for not running away when we got to the "for worse" part in our marriage. Thank you for keeping me, even though I turned out to be a real fixer-upper!

Bryn, for making me laugh, cry, and sometimes both at the same time! I adore you; you are perfect exactly as you are. Never change. I love you THIS much!

Dana, my angel baby, for always seeing the good in people. You remind me every day why it is wonderful to be alive. You are beautiful inside and out. "I love you all day long."

My dad, Don, and step-mom, Dot, for seamlessly stepping in to help every single time I need you; sometimes before I even realize I need you. Thanks for propping us all up in spite of your own pain, and for reminding me to let go and let God.

My sister, Shelley (Bug) Welstead, who is more than a sister and greater than a best friend, for simply making my life better every day that she is in it. There is no greater security net than you. I am proud of who you are and of the life you are living. Thank you for taking such good care of me. I'm happy to share a brain with you!

My soul sister, Tanya (LaRue) Noye, my best friend, for always saying the right thing at the perfect time. We met to make each other's lives better and I thank God for you everyday. *"You complete me." (wink)*

My "Katie", (Kate Devine), for your deep, unconditional love. You know me better than I know myself.

Cathy (Stark) Pearce, for always "getting me"and for being a friend I can always count on. "Ooh, baby I like the sound when..."

My Chatham family, for joining forces with the Adams clan and supporting me through it all.

Linda Lazier, for your enthusiastic support. Thank you for believing in me.

Suzanne Welstead, my sister in law and fellow writer, for sharing the "first book" experience with me. I thank God every day that you came along.

My grandma, Rachael Forestell. You are everyone's favourite family member! Everything we know about strength and dignity in the face of hardship we learned from your example.

Acknowledgements

My Other Glove, Susan LeRue, for always fitting just right. Your warmth has gotten me through many cold spells.

My survivor friends: Mary, Lee, Bonnie, Sandi, Carol, Bambi, Sandra, Donna, Jenn Maidens, the Guelph Breaststrokes Dragon Boat team, The Guelph Breast Cancer Support Group, and in loving memory of Kim Walker and Dianne Yates.

My mom, Nancy Adams, for teaching me how to be a mother and friend, how to laugh, and for sharing with me the joy that can only be found in the written word. I miss you.

About the Author

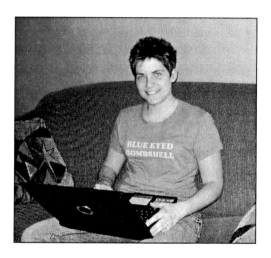

Marcie Nolan is a writer, motivational public speaker, and elementary school teacher living in Guelph, Ontario, with her husband, Jeff, and their two daughters, Bryn and Dana. Marcie is a breast cancer survivor who believes in using the power of humour to overcome life's obstacles. Marcie's website www.headonastick.ca will soon be available for more information.

$1 from each book sold will be donated
to the Juravinski Cancer Centre in Hamilton, Ontario